YOUR GUIDE TO MODERN PLASTIC SURGERY

HOW TO ENHANCE YOUR NATURAL BEAUTY AND AVOID A PLASTIC SURGERY DISASTER

Dr Laith Barnouti, FRACS (Plastic)
Specialist Plastic Surgeon

TABLE OF CONTENTS

FOREWORD

It is a pleasure to write a few words about Dr Barnouti's book, *Your Guide to Modern Plastic Surgery*. Laith visited us in Gent, Belgium in 2009 for a three-month period as a young plastic surgeon travelling around the world visiting different renowned and established plastic surgery departments. Already then, his special interest in aesthetic surgery was obvious.

I remember him as a very enjoyable, intelligent and sharp-minded young plastic surgeon. I was sure he would find his way and build up a beautiful career in the Wild West of plastic surgery. In aesthetic surgery, what you see is important, but even more important is what you don't see.

Laith was one of those surgeons who had interest in these small details that just make all the difference. I remember him questioning me during surgeries, as I normally do not talk much while I am operating. But instead of annoying me, he amused me with his sharp and detailed search for what he wanted to learn.

I remember answering his questions for which I did not know the answer by telling him: "The secret ingredient is always love!" Reading the book that Laith just wrote, I am glad to see that he incorporated this philosophy into his work.

The reason Dr Barnouti wrote this book is not to add more patients to his busy working schedule. He wrote it because he is passionate about his work. He loves what he is doing. He loves to help patients in their struggle against ageing or being disfigured from birth or following trauma or weight loss. Being an aesthetic surgeon for the last 30 years, I know how an aesthetic intervention can change a patient's life so thoroughly. The gratitude of these patients is so overwhelming that I consider plastic surgery as one of the most mentally rewarding and interesting professions ever.

I am glad and proud that Laith has become who he is now, that he became an expert in his field, that he built up a beautiful family and that he did not forget "that the secret ingredient is always love…"

Patrick Tonnard, MD, PhD
SPECIALIST PLASTIC SURGEON
GENT, BELGIUM
SEPTEMBER 2019

———○———

AUTHOR'S NOTE

This book marks more than 20 years since I started my surgical training at the Queen Elizabeth Hospital in South Australia and more than 15 years of practising in the field of plastic surgery.

In 2008, I was granted my fellowship of the Royal Australasian College of Surgeons, FRACS (Plastic).

In 2020, I was invited to become a Conjoint Lecturer in medicine and surgery at the University of New South Wales and from July 2022 I have been a Conjoint Senior Lecturer.

I have travelled the world seeking more knowledge, answers and experience in plastic surgery. My international fellowship training was in Rio De Janeiro (Brazil), Stockholm (Sweden) and Gent (Belgium). I feel privileged to have trained with some of the best surgeons in the world. It opened my mind and widened my knowledge.

These last 15 years plus of running plastic surgery clinics in Sydney hold an excellent record of safety. I provide my patients with the best possible care and aesthetic outcomes. This includes delivering surgery in a meticulous manner and not ignoring the vital post-operative and recovery phases.

I am also very open and honest with patients. Every week, I send patients away; telling them they don't need surgery.

Patients are often surprised when they are told by a specialist plastic surgeon that surgery is not recommended for them. Surgery needs to be performed for the right reasons. I remind patients every day that surgery is trauma to the body in a controlled manner.

I am not in the business of "selling surgery". Rather I pride myself in providing the best health advice to my patients and putting their health first and foremost. As a medical practitioner, I have taken the Hippocratic Oath to "do no harm".

While plastic surgery can be very satisfying by bringing happiness to patients and changing their lives, I take this profession very seriously. I hold a great deal of responsibility because patients trust me with their health.

This is done through careful consultation and communication. Planning for surgery will only be put in place if I feel it is in the patient's best interests.

Finally, it's important to mention that all the "before and after" photos in this book are of patients who I have operated on during the last 15 years. None have been altered or Photoshopped.

Enjoy the book.

Dr Laith Barnouti
SPECIALIST PLASTIC SURGEON, FRACS
CONJOINT SENIOR LECTURER, UNIVERSITY OF NSW
SYDNEY, AUSTRALIA
AUGUST 2024

ACKNOWLEDGMENTS

Many thanks to my beautiful and original wife, Dr Zoe Potres and my three amazing children Lara, Lydia and Oscar. You keep me grounded.

I would like to acknowledge the support of my energetic and enthusiastic father, Dr Ramzi Barnouti OAM and my mother, Hannah, who is always keen to know what I am doing and if I am busy enough with my work!

I am grateful to have been brought up as a member of the medical "Barnouti" family who emphasise achievements, hard work and ethics. They have provided me with guidance, love and support along the way.

With a special mention to my mentors in the plastic surgery field: Dr Patrick Tonnard (Belgium), Dr Per Heden (Sweden), the late Professor Ivo Pitanguy (Brazil), Dr Alex Verpaele (Belgium), Dr Daniel Baker (USA), Dr Michael Poole (Australia), Dr Michael Baldwin (Australia), Dr David Pennington (Australia) and Dr Paul Curtin (Australia).

ACKNOWLEDGMENTS

I consider myself lucky to have worked with some of the best surgeons in the world and learned their techniques, ethics and commitment to work.

I would like to thank my work partner and skilled surgeon, Dr Mark Kohout, for a great working relationship throughout the years. We run and manage one of the most successful plastic surgery clinics in Australia. It is a partnership that is based on trust and respect. We share not only knowledge and ideas, but also great responsibilities in always attempting to deliver the best standard of care and aesthetic outcomes for our patients.

A successful practice requires mature, dedicated and committed staff. I have been lucky enough to have worked with great anaesthetists, surgical assistants, registrars and nurses. All made possible by an exceptional personal assistant, Jessie Elliot. Thank you.

I would like to acknowledge the staff at Westmead Private, Hunters Hill Private, City West Specialist and Sydney Private hospitals for providing a safe environment and great facilities for my patients.

And finally, to my patients who keep me intellectually motivated by seeking answers to different problems... this book is for you.

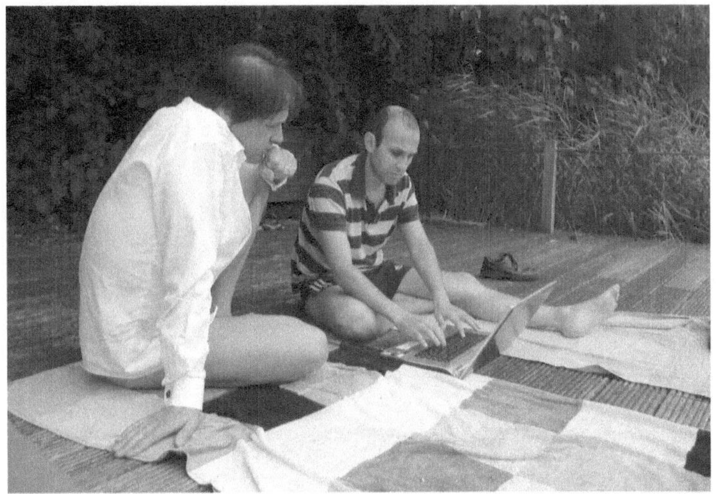

Here is a view into my private life as I write a plastic surgery paper with Dr Patrick Tonnard next to a private lake in Gent, Belgium.

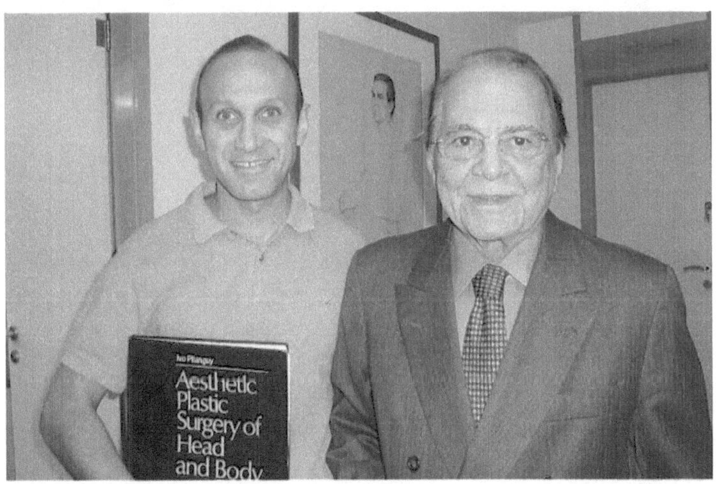

Dr Laith Barnouti in Rio De Janeiro with the father of modern plastic surgery, Professor Ivo Pitanguy. "I feel privileged to have worked and learned from the Master of the trade," says Dr Barnouti of Prof Pitanguy who died in 2016.

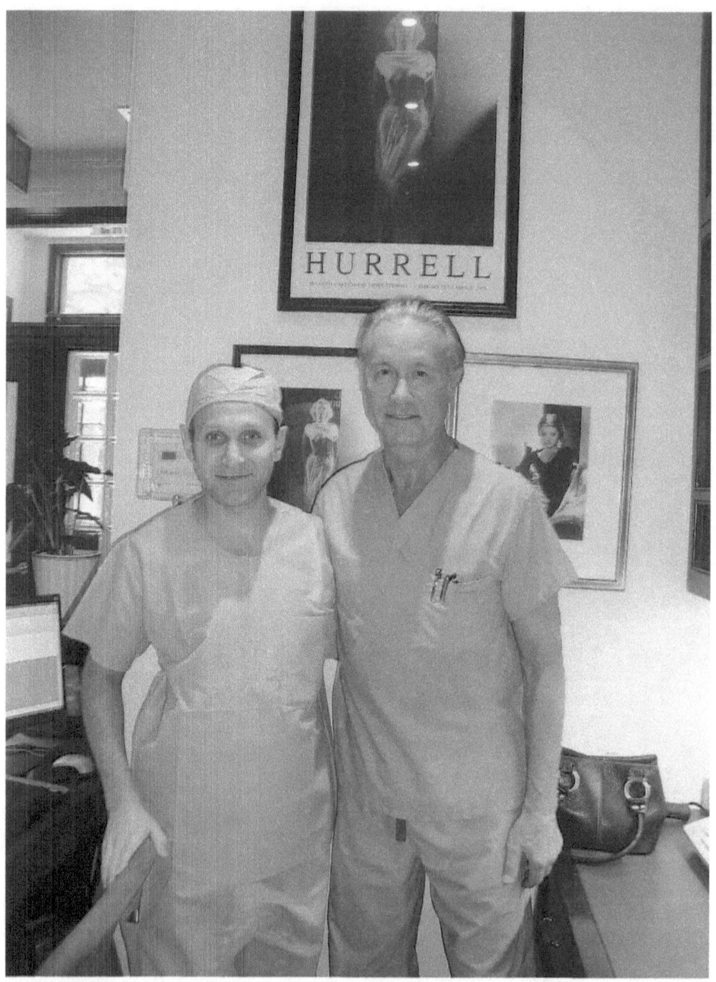

In New York with Dr Daniel Baker. "He broadened my knowledge of facial plastic surgery."

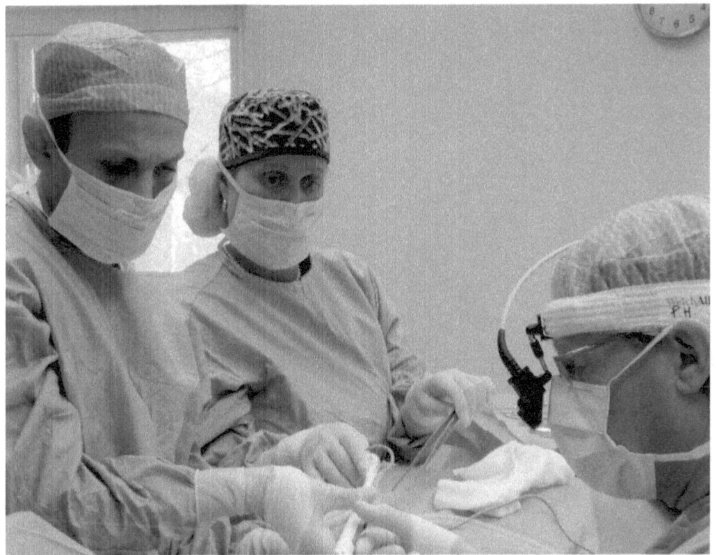

Dr Laith Barnouti at Akademikliniken Plastikkirurgi, Sweden's largest plastic surgery clinic, performing breast surgery with Dr Per Heden. Dr Barnouti spent three months in Stockholm, Sweden perfecting his skills in breast surgery.

INTRODUCTION

wanted my outer appearance to match how I felt on the inside," says Claudia, events coordinator at a four-star hotel in Sydney.

"I never felt as old as my calendar age, but there's no doubt my wisdom and experience were starting to really show. My industry is dominated by men, and I was getting tired of being passed over for promotions. It became obvious that looks count. It is sad, but it is reality – like it or not. And even putting aside my professional goals, I was tired of looking tired."

This is what prompted Claudia to have her plastic surgery.

Over my years as a plastic surgeon, I have heard the same story from so many patients. They hate it when their family and friends tag them in Facebook photos. Some of them find themselves staring into the mirror and pulling their neck or facial skin back or lifting their cheeks.

Are you one of them? Do you hate your droopy jowls? Do you look like you aren't getting enough sleep? What about that little nose hump that you wish you didn't have? What about your stubborn body fat that isn't responding to diet and exercise? Do you feel that pregnancy or weight fluctuation may have affected your tummy, breast or genital areas? Do these problem areas make you feel less attractive and confident?

How confident you feel is often tied to your physical appearance. Unfortunately, there is very little you can do personally to change a part of the body or face you were born with – or how it changes as you age and are exposed to physiological or pathological changes.

You may have wrestled with the notion of having plastic surgery but are still not sure. You don't want to end up looking like one of those over-the-top plastic surgery disasters, who have achieved the opposite of the desired effect by drawing attention to their age. But at the same time, you may see or know people who you admire for the successful "work" they have had done, because they look more vibrant than they did before.

It's no secret that plastic surgery can help you achieve what you want for your face and/or body.

So, if you want the confidence that comes from looking your best, then *Your Guide to Modern Plastic Surgery* is for you. It focusses on the positive change in your appearance that can be achieved safely by plastic surgery when performed by expert hands.

I explain the wide range of surgical and non-surgical options available to you, what realistic results you can hope to achieve and ultimately, how your life can be drastically changed.

This book isn't only for women!

While women make up the majority of my patients, men are increasingly choosing to use plastic surgery to enhance their facial features and sculpt their bodies.

Robert, a retail salesperson, chose to pursue a facelift. His reasons were a little different to my previous patient, Claudia:

I had my facelift at the age of 58 because my looks were not a reflection of me. I've always been an athlete, and my body still looks great, but my face started heading south when I was in my forties. Every year I felt more droopy and tired looking. I also felt my job opportunities would be better if I looked fresher and healthier. Plastic surgery took 10 years off my face and neck, and now I look more vibrant.

While their goals were different, Claudia and Robert share a common theme of wanting to feel happier about themselves.

The good news is that the surgical and non-surgical options highlighted in this book are no longer the exclusive domain of celebrities. Plastic surgery has become more affordable throughout the years because of the increased number of surgical options and providers as well as the availability of payment plan options.

If other methods, such as diet and exercise, haven't yielded the results you want, then consider other options such as plastic surgery. Your specialist plastic surgeon will outline any possible risks of undergoing surgery and provide advice as to whether cosmetic surgery is for you or not.

The cultural shift in this age of social media can sometimes force people to become "too obsessed" with their appearance.

While cosmetic surgery can improve and enhance your face and body, a "perfect outcome" is both unrealistic and unachievable.

If you're looking for "perfection", remember that perfection is unattainable. The human body is naturally asymmetrical, and it can be even more beautiful for its asymmetry.

I remind patients that surgery has limitations and that some surgical procedures may not be in their best interests. However, usually there are real solutions available that will rejuvenate and improve your looks as well as boosting your confidence.

CHAPTER ONE

Face and Neck

First impressions are everything, and your face can send the wrong message.

Frown lines, saggy skin, deep wrinkles and droopy eyes can broadcast to the world, "I'm tired, stressed out and unhappy". Even if you don't feel that way, it's what people see.

You may be genetically predisposed to certain types of ageing, and no amount of proper diet, exercise or even avoiding the sun can prevent the way your face ages.

If you want to feel younger and healthier and you want your face to reflect your inner glow, then plastic surgery can offer you a range of surgical and non-surgical solutions.

Nose Surgery

Sandra always disliked her profile. For someone with otherwise delicate facial features, she felt as though her Roman nose belonged on another face. She had casually started considering a nose job but wasn't sure if she had the guts to change her appearance. However, Sandra also suffered from obstructed breathing because of a deviated septum. Since she needed to correct her deviated septum anyway, Sandra ultimately decided to have a procedure that would improve her breathing as well as change the shape of her nose to something more proportionate to her face. Sandra's septo-rhinoplasty operation (improvement in nose shape and breathing) gave her the functionality and the looks that she was hoping for. Her only regret was waiting until she was 35 to have it done!

The desire for a different nose shape is one of the most common reasons people choose plastic surgery. This type of operation is broadly called rhinoplasty because "rhino" means nose. Some patients wish to reduce or increase the size of their nose, change the shape of the tip or the bridge, narrow the span of their nostrils, or change the angle between their nose and upper lip.

One of the most popular procedures is rhinoplasty. It involves reshaping of the nose to make it smaller, straighter and in proportion with other facial structures. A skillful plastic surgeon will produce a natural-looking nose, which is in harmony with the patient's other facial features.

This is achieved through careful planning and a full understanding of facial anatomy. Excess cartilage and bone are removed, allowing the natural skin envelope to shrink down to the smaller framework. My main objective in this procedure is to produce a smaller, natural-looking nose and improve or maintain the patient's breathing capacity.

Some patients, such as Asian patients, require an augmentation rhinoplasty technique to enlarge the nose. This procedure uses either natural tissue or a nasal implant to create a nose that will match the patient's facial and racial characteristics. **See Chapter 7: Asian Plastic Surgery.**

The skin of the nose has no shape; it is the underlying cartilage and bony architecture that provide shape. Therefore, smaller noses require precise placement of grafts from the patient's own tissue and sometimes implant material (such as silicone, Gortex or Medpore) to produce a natural-looking nose.

Some patients are happy with the size of their noses but not with the shape. Reshaping rhinoplasty may focus on the shape of the tip, the bridge or the root of the nose. Reshaping rhinoplasty can be addressed with a variety of procedures ranging from a simple non-invasive technique to a larger scale surgical procedure. Finally, some patients

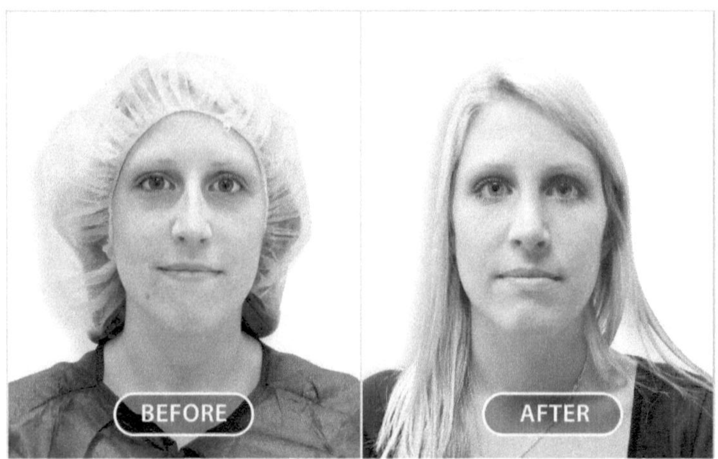

Both the front and side views are equally appealing, while her breathing functionality is improved.

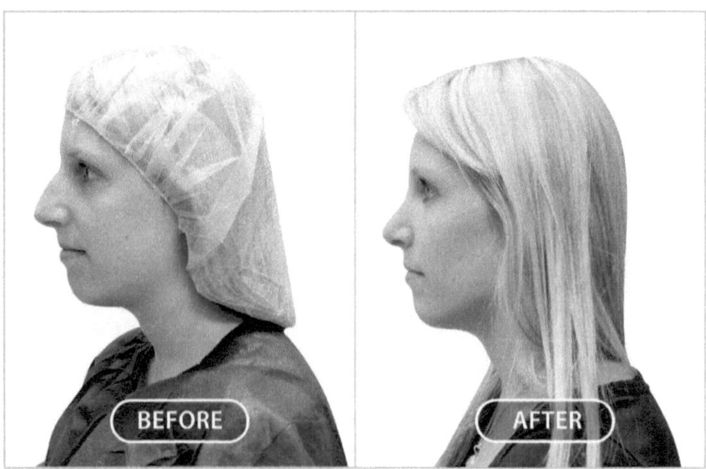

require work on their airway, and this can be achieved by performing a combined septo-rhinoplasty and turbinate reduction (the turbinate is an anatomical structure situated inside the nose that may become enlarged for a number of reasons). The surgery results in a pleasing shape and increased functionality of the nose, as demonstrated by improved breathing. Decision making happens after careful consideration. Some patients will benefit from "closed rhinoplasty," where the surgery is performed from inside the nose with no visible outside scars. Others will be more suitable for "open rhinoplasty", which involves an 8 mm incision in the columella (the vertical strip of tissue separating the nostrils) to lift the nose skin, so the procedure is done under direct vision.

A few patients who visit plastic surgeons require only septoplasty, or the correction of a deviated septum. In this procedure, the septum is straightened, meaning the deviated part of the septum is removed to open both airways and ensure easy breathing through both nostrils.

The initial consultation allows me to determine whether a patient is suitable for a "soft treatment" or whether a surgical solution is required. I can provide a soft treatment, such as filler to augment the nose, on the same day as the consultation.

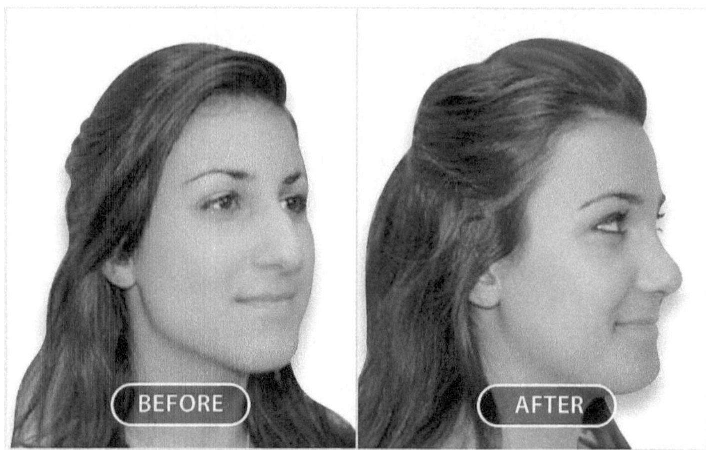

The final nose shape is in harmony with the rest of the facial features.

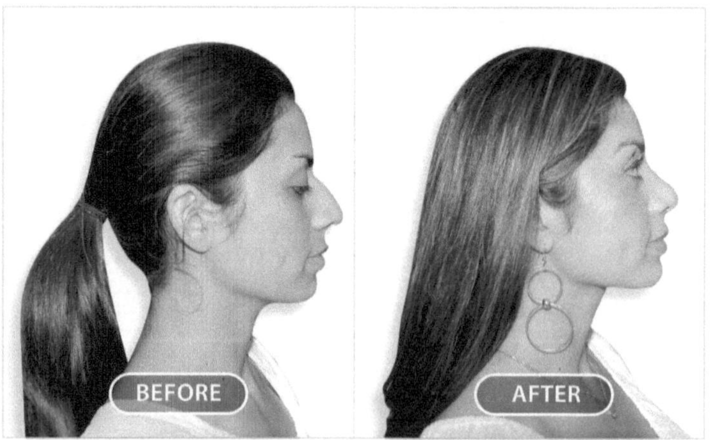

Septo-rhinoplasty and turbinate reduction work together to improve breathing.

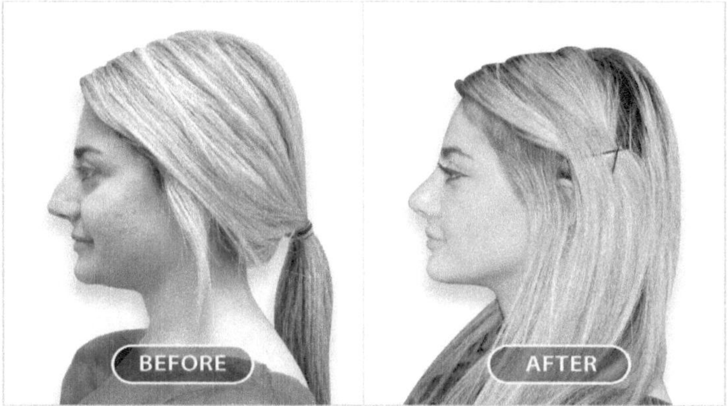

A natural-looking rhinoplasty result, with additional acne scar treatment.

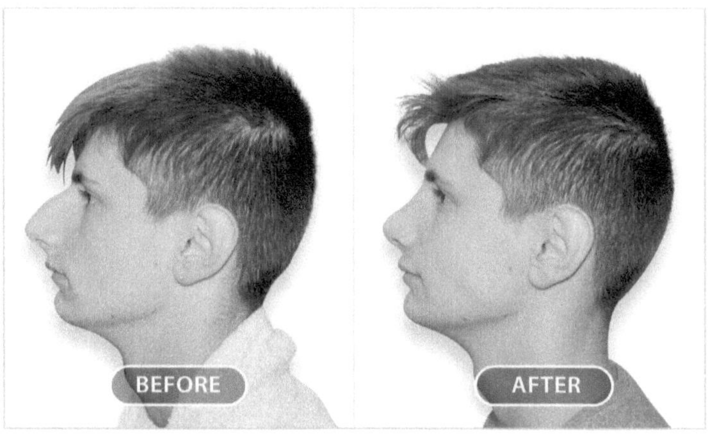

Men's noses should not appear or look too small. It will not suit the face and will look disproportional.

Facelift

I had always looked younger than my calendar years. I saw my good plastic surgeon when I was 45, and he said, "You are too young for a facelift, and you should consider instead minimally invasive techniques such as laser resurfacing with fat/stem cells injection".

Then, as I journeyed through my fifties, age and sun damage started to catch up with me. Looking in the mirror, I just didn't recognise the woman in the mirror compared to how felt inside. My facial skin was saggy and crepey. I would ask myself, who IS that old woman?

Finally, when I reached 58, I'd had enough. Given my age and facial characteristics, my surgeon recommended I go for a full face, neck and temporal lift, eyelid surgery and laser resurfacing. Yes – "the works"!

The recovery was not as hard as I expected. I struggled with the bandage around my head for a couple of days, but it was fine afterwards. I feel 15 years younger, and most importantly, I look natural. My laugh lines are softer. My crepey skin is gone. I look like I'm happy and awake. I still have a face with expressions, and I love what I see in the mirror!

~ Darlene G.

As we age, most people lose the youthful volume in the mid-face region. The appearance of wrinkles or deep lines close to the eyelids or around the mouth and other visible signs of ageing can be successfully corrected with a face and neck lift, which is medically known as a rhytidectomy.

I customise my procedure to each patient using the latest facial rejuvenation and facelift techniques, which involve much more than simply tightening the skin and deep tissue. My comprehensive facial strategy is designed specifically to recreate a youthful appearance in the face, neck, eyelids, temporal and forehead areas.

Surgery may include skin resurfacing, targeted liposuction, volumetric restoration, such as fat injection, laser, a TCA peel, and other complementary surgical procedures that result in a natural, youthful appearance.

My face and neck lift strategies are based on the importance of shifting facial volumes rather than old-fashioned facelift techniques, which just pull back the skin. Restoration of facial volumes is more important than the amount of skin that is surgically removed.

Facial rejuvenation and facial recontouring are two different approaches, with different outcomes. Facial rejuvenation is for those who want to look 10–15 years younger (the majority of my patients). Facial recontouring creates significant facial changes and is not commonly requested.

Within these categories, I tailor the procedure based on the patient's needs, as follows:

- Mini facelift – is sometimes called a Hollywood facelift. This procedure involves a small incision in the hairline only. Recovery time is two-to-five days and the resulting scar is unnoticeable as it will be hidden, covered by the hair.

- Short scar facelift – also known as an S lift or MACS lift. The incision is made at the junction of the ear and the side of the cheek but finishes at the earlobe and does not extend behind the ear. The recovery time is five-to-eight days and there will be no scar behind the ear.

- Full face and neck lift – also known as an SMAS face and neck lift. The incision is at the junction of the ear and cheek and behind the ear, creating what is known as an omega scar. This is a longer and more extensive procedure with a recovery time of eight-to-14 days.

- Total facial rejuvenation – this includes a facelift, neck lift, fat transfer, temporal lift, liplift, skin resurfacing by laser or chemical peel, and upper and lower blepharoplasty (eyelid surgery).

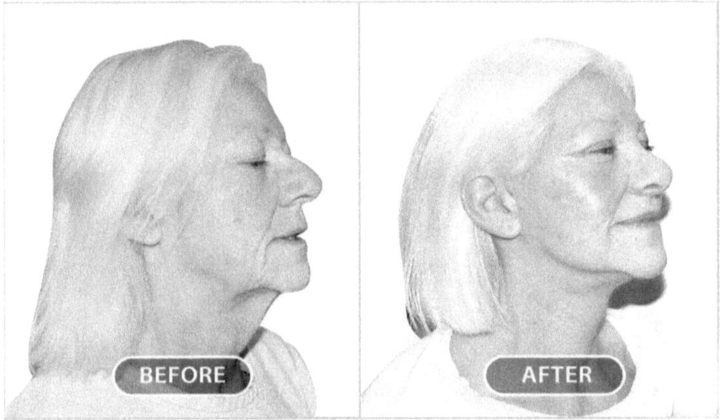

A facelift and necklift results in a natural, youthful appearance.

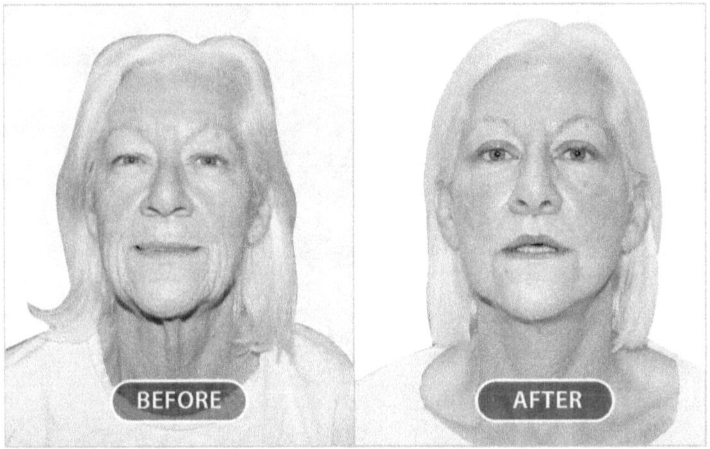

The key for successful face and neck surgery is to rejuvenate the face, turning the clock back 10–15 years and maintaining the same features. We do not need to change an individual's features. We only need to refresh and rejuvenate them.

Full face rejuvenation surgery can be performed under general anaesthetic and takes around four hours depending on the extent of the procedure.

With most facelifts, after making the incision, I separate the skin from the fat and muscle below. Fat may be trimmed or liposuctioned from around the neck and chin to improve the contour of the face. I then tighten the underlying muscles and membranes. Volume is usually added to certain areas such as the cheekbones for enhancement.

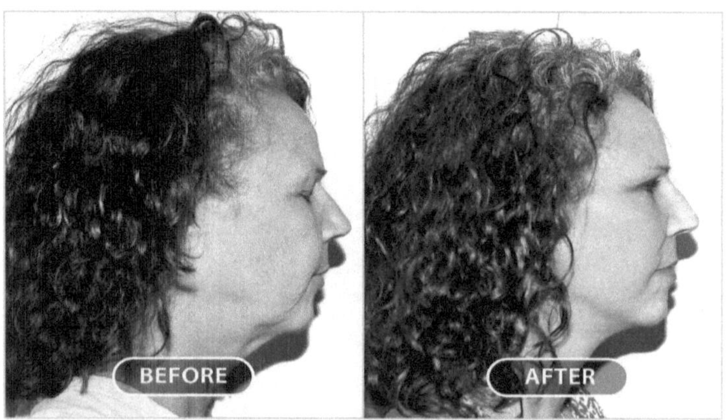

Shifting facial volumes creates amazing results.

Other complementary procedures may also be undertaken to achieve the best possible results:

- Eyelid surgery on the upper and/or lower eyelids, also known as blepharoplasty;

- Neck lift, neck liposuction and recontouring;

- Brow lift;

- Lip lift, augmentation, resurfacing or combination;

- Tear trough procedure to improve on the appearance of a displeasing under-eye groove;

- Cheekbone enhancement with fat transfer or cheek implants;

- Smoothening the nasolabial folds and marionette lines (smile lines);

- Nose reshaping or rhinoplasty;

- Chin reshaping;

- Laser treatment;

- Soft treatments;

- Lipofilling, fat injection;

All incisions are closed using fine sutures, so they do not leave marks when they are removed.

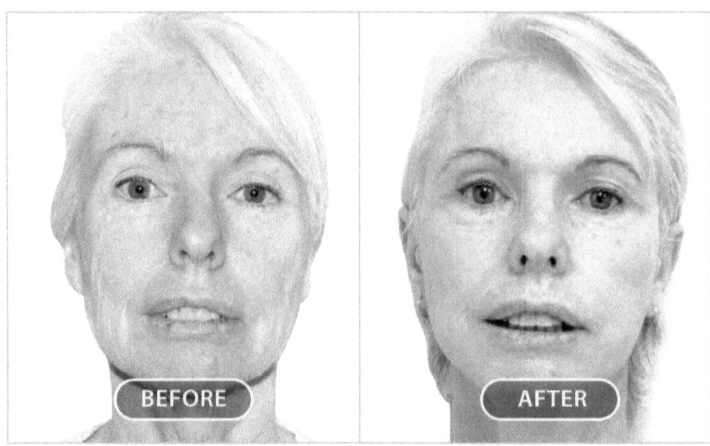

This patient had neck and facelift surgery.

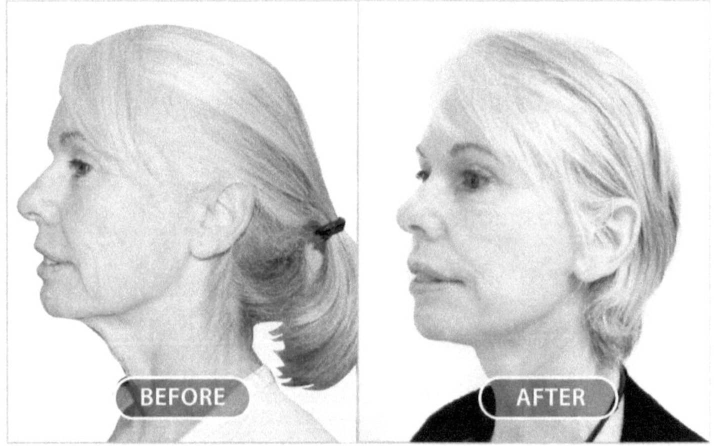

Youthful appearance and better definition of jaw line.

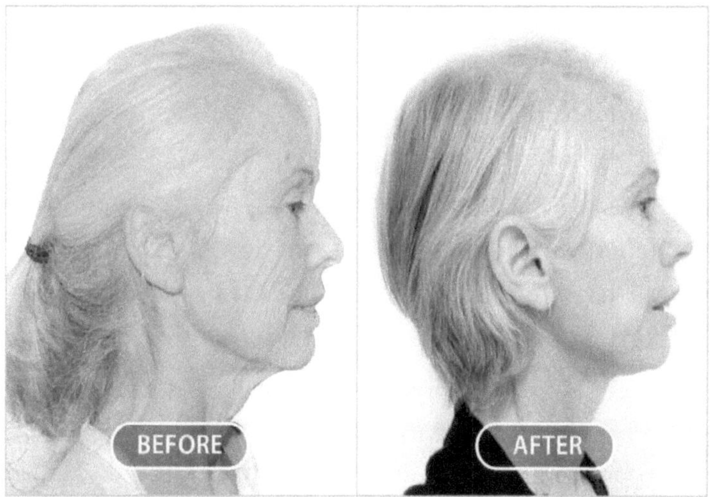

You can see where the volume was added, enhancing this patient's cheekbones.

Brow Lift

"I feel like my face is melting," Angela once told her best friend. She recalls how she brought her fingertips to the outer edges of her eyebrows and slid them up toward her hair. "My eyebrows used to be up here," Angela told her friend, "and now I look like a sad puppy." She then moved her fingers away from her face, and her brows slid back down to their droopy position, which partially obscured the outer corners of her deep blue eyes. After careful consultation, Angela decided to improve her appearance with a facial plastic surgery procedure called a brow and temporal lift. The brow/temporal lift raised her eyebrows, got rid of the sad droopy look, smoothed her forehead and eliminated her scowl lines.

A fullness of the brow, upper eyelid and the temple region is fundamental for a healthy, youthful and sensual appearance. As the fullness of youth disappears, the structures underneath emerge. In the upper face, the shape of the skull and the rims around the eyes become more prominent. The blood vessels are no longer concealed by fullness and become more visible. With ageing, the muscles of facial expressions are more noticeable, the eyebrows descend, the eyes become more deep-set and skeletal, and many older people wear a permanent frown or scowl.

The lack of fullness results in an empty sac of skin sagging where the fullness was previously present.

Through the "structural microfat grafting" technique that I use as a synergistic procedure in a brow lift, I restore the brow and forehead area to more youthful and healthy proportions by replacing the fatty tissue that has atrophied through the years.

A brow lift – sometimes called a temporal or forehead lift – improves lateral hooding (the droopy flaps of skin that hang over the outside corner of the eyes). Plastic surgery of the forehead will also soften horizontal forehead wrinkles and scowl lines between the eyebrows for a more youthful appearance.

The upper half of the face ages one decade before the lower half; therefore, the upper half is typically operated on first.

A brow lift is performed through a 5 cm incision located at the top of the head behind or in line with the hairline to hide the final scar. The skin and fascia on the head, brow and around the eyes will be raised and set in a higher position. This approach naturally rejuvenates the upper eyelids and brow area. The procedure takes about 60 minutes and the patient can go home the same day as the procedure.

I recommend that my patients have this procedure performed in combination with fat injections and/or laser resurfacing to treat deep forehead wrinkle lines.

Eyelid Surgery

A couple of years ago, I was getting ready for my daughter's engagement party. I remember thinking to myself, "What's the point of putting on makeup?" My upper eyelids were drooping to the point that they had started to affect my vision. The eyelid bags underneath looked like half-filled saggy water balloons. I looked like a bloodhound.

I put on my big sunglasses and went to the party, feeling much older than my 46 years. The wedding would be six months later, and so I thought that I had better do something about it now.

I didn't want to turn back time. I like my laugh lines. Every wrinkle tells a story. But those eyes! My eyelids made me look 20 older!

The day following the engagement party, I booked a consultation to find out what I could do and opted for eyelid surgery. I had upper and lower blepharoplasty (top and bottom eyelid surgery) to lift my eyelids and get rid of those awful bags under my eyes. The results were amazing. I had people approach me at Caitlin's wedding asking me if I was Caitlin's sister!

~ Carmen A.

Eyelid surgery, which is also called upper and lower blepharoplasty, is an effective way to correct droopy eyelids, bags under the eyes, puffy eyelids and/or under-eye sagging. The procedure recontours and reshapes the upper and/or lower eyelids by trimming away excess skin and fat from the eye area to create a more youthful appearance.

Close attention needs to be paid to the pre-operative condition of the eyelids, surrounding tissue and bone structure to create a natural appearance and prevent an "operated-on look". Removal of excess skin and fatty tissue will tighten the eyelids and restore an attractive almond shape to the eyes while meticulous attention to surgical detail can avoid a "hollowed" appearance or unwanted complications.

Ancillary procedures can be performed at the same time as eyelid surgery to optimise the outcome. These include: laser, fat injection, a brow lift and/or facelift.

In a typical eyelid plastic surgery procedure, an incision is made in the natural line of the upper eyelids, normally in the creases of the upper eyelids.

Incisions for lower eyelid surgery are made just below the eyelashes or inside the conjunctiva, which is the inner surface of the eyelid. Working through these incisions, the skin is separated from the underlying fatty tissue and muscle. The excess fat bulges are then removed and transposed (rearranged). If required, I trim away any sagging skin and muscle. The incisions are then closed with very fine sutures, and the final scar is virtually undetectable six weeks after surgery.

Upper Eyelid Surgery

With the ageing process, the skin of the upper eyelid tends to sag. This is not only aesthetically displeasing but also makes one appear older. In severe cases, it places gravitational pressure on the eyelashes, obscuring vision and making the eyes look and feel tired.

Upper eyelid surgery to remove excess upper eyelid skin is a delicate operation. During this 60-minute procedure, the excess skin is trimmed, the saggy portion of the muscle is excised or tightened and the fat bulges removed. Sutures are removed after seven days.

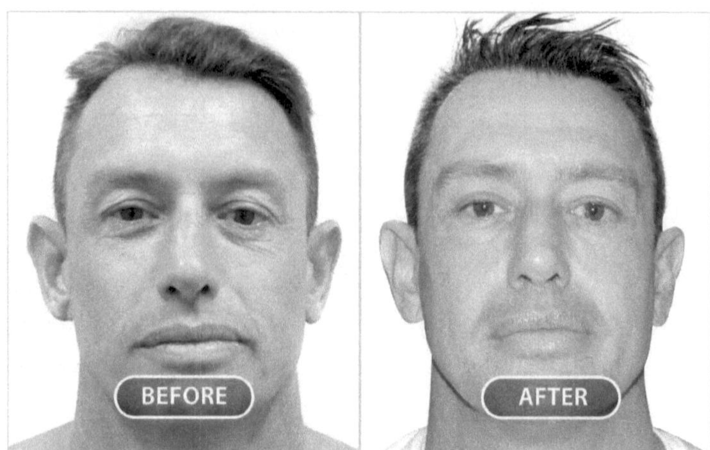

Upper eyelid surgery performed with laser rejuvenation. Notice the improvement in the skin quality of the lower eyelids without direct surgery to the lower eyelids. It is often a bonus to have lower eyelids skin improvement when performing upper blepharoplasty, provided a lateral tunnel has been created for blood pooling.

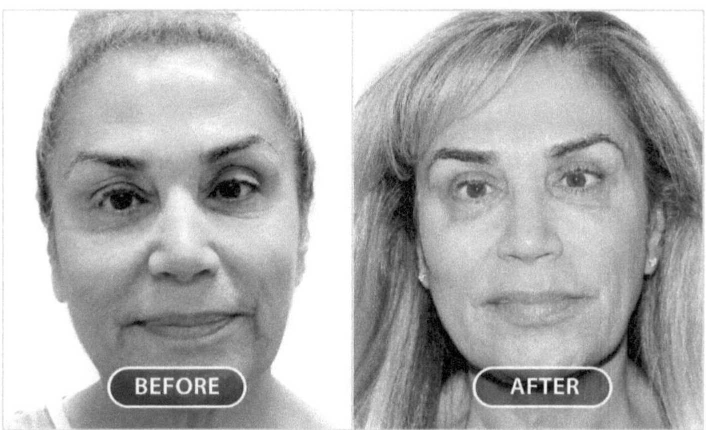

When I perform upper eyelid surgery, I create a tunnel to the lower eyelids in the most lateral part of my incision. This reduces the risk of pre-septal haematoma. A small amount of blood trickles into the lower eyelids, producing a PRP effect. Notice the slight improvement in the lower eyelids, even though I have not operated on the lower eyelids.

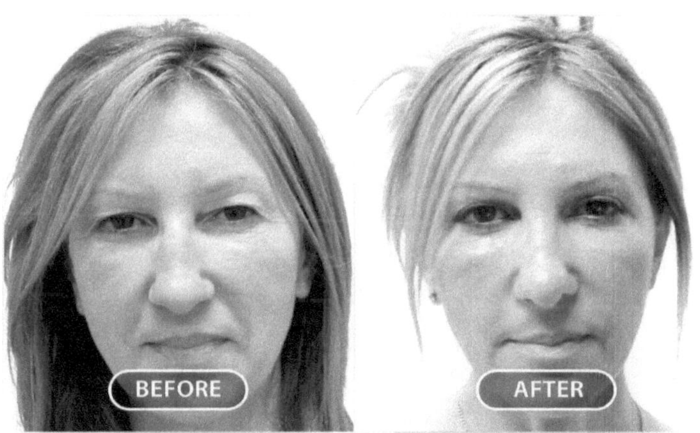

This is the result of upper eyelid surgery. Notice the slight improvement to the lower eyelids even though I have not operated on the lower eyelids. A plasma rich protein effect through a lateral tunnel.

Lower Eyelid Surgery

The presence of lower eyelid bags can often indicate the person is overworked, tired or the ageing process is starting to take its toll. For this reason, many patients decide that they want to change what their eyes say about them by opting to have lower eyelid surgery.

Different types of incision are made with lower eyelid surgery. The most common is the subcilliary, in which the incision is made just underneath the line of the lash. This approach is used when the skin is loose and requires removal in addition to the removal of the bulging fat pads.

If there's a pocket of fat underneath the lower eyelids, but there is no loose skin to be removed, then the preferable approach is a transconjunctival one where an incision is made on the inside of the lower eyelid with no external scar. This approach is often used in conjunction with laser treatment to rejuvenate the lower eyelid skin.

The objective of this delicate surgery is to smooth out the bulges, remove the bags from underneath the eyes and make the skin snugger.

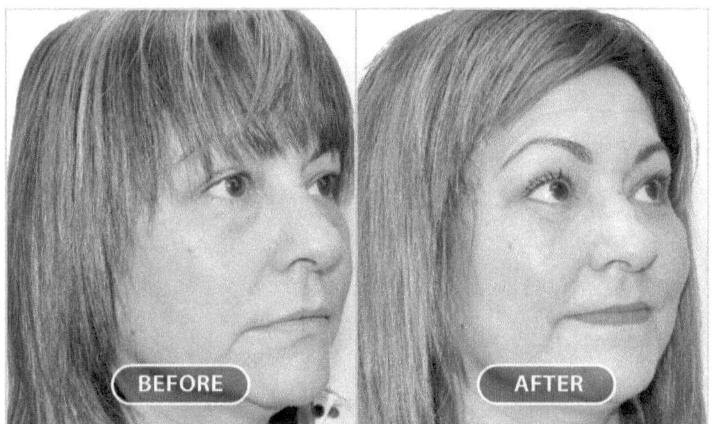

Removal and redrapping of lower eyelid fat bags through an internal transconjunctival incision. The key point is to avoid excess fat removal as it will produce undesirable hallowing.

Lazy Eyelid Surgery

Some people are born with lazy eyelids and some develop the condition later in life. Either way, a "droopy eyelid" or "lazy eyelid" gives one an appearance of looking sleepy and unfocused. The reason for a droopy eyelid is a functional weakness of the eyelid-opening mechanism, called the levator.

Lazy eyelid surgery, sometimes called ptosis correction surgery, corrects these droopy eyes by tightening the levator muscle. It is a very delicate procedure and should only be performed by experienced specialist plastic surgeons.

Fat Injection Surgery

Linda is an architect and a passionate surfer. She had always been puzzled by something her German grandmother used to say: "As you get older, your face will either become that of a goat, or that of a cow". Linda didn't understand this amusing saying until she reached her forties. She had always had a long, narrow face.

One morning as she walked to meet a friend for coffee, Linda saw her reflection in a shop window. "I look good", she thought, noticing her fit, lean body. But then she noticed a dramatic shadow under her cheekbones. Her cheeks were sunken and hollow. Linda didn't have a lot of wrinkles and her skin tone was good; however, her cheeks had lost all of their fullness.

Linda realised with a shock, "I look like a goat!"

Over the years, Linda's cheeks had become sunken, almost skeletonised, as the plumpness of her cheeks was replaced with deep shadows. This sunken appearance made her feel old. Linda saw me and expressed her desire for a more youthful appearance. I suggested that I widen the upper and mid part of her face, augment (plump up) her cheeks, and effectively transform her face from long and narrow to a wide triangular shape with the best filler in the world, her own fat.

This is a procedure known as lipofilling or fat injection surgery. The cheek, midface, temporal and forehead fat injections have transformed Linda's face, restored volume and produced a proportional face. Linda looks younger and healthier; a look that reflects her inner vitality and energy.

As we age and lose volume and the plumpness of youth, our faces literally become smaller. The skin remains the same size, but without the underlying structure, it retreats into wrinkles. Fat injections diminish wrinkles as the lost structure under the skin is restored.

Since shrinkage of the subcutaneous tissues is the key sign of ageing, replacement of the atrophied tissue with a technique called "structural microfat grafting" is the best method of facial rejuvenation. Diffusely augmenting (plumping) the structure of the forehead, cheeks, mouth, chin and jaw line restores the fullness of youth.

Traditional cosmetic surgery procedures have tried to eliminate wrinkles, bags, jowls and folds. Unfortunately, they do not take into account how people looked when they were younger. Consequently, the end result of a facelift or eye tuck is that while the person may be tighter, they do not look like they did when they were young, simply because sufficient facial fat is no longer present. With few exceptions, traditional plastic surgery revolves around a single solution to the challenges of augmentation and rejuvenation – cutting away fat/skin and tightening the muscle.

The 21st-century approach to advanced plastic surgery pays specific attention to supporting vital structures and volumetric restoration of the face and body with living filler (the patient's own fat), correcting asymmetry and restoring the fullness of youth, naturally and subtly. It is important to know that eliminating wrinkles alone does not necessarily create a youthful appearance; the secret lies in replacing fullness to a face.

Structural microfat grafting (fat injection) is a revolutionary technique that uses the patient's own body fat as a natural, living filler to achieve precise structural alterations wherever it is placed. It is safe, adaptable and undetectable. Transplanted fat that originates from the patient does not carry a risk of allergic reaction or rejection. Further advantages include a short recovery time, no scars and long-lasting results.

Structural micro fat grafting reinstates the fullness lost due to ageing and can be used to rejuvenate and enhance all areas of the face including the chin, nose, neck, jawline, nasolabial folds, marionette lines, brow, upper eyelids, temples, lips, breasts, buttocks and areas of the lower body. It can correct deformities, such as hemifacial atrophy, problems caused by previous liposuction, and also cleft palate. Fat grafting is presently being used as an ancillary procedure to a facelift, brow lift, blepharoplasty, rhinoplasty, eyelid surgery, forehead lift and breast augmentation.

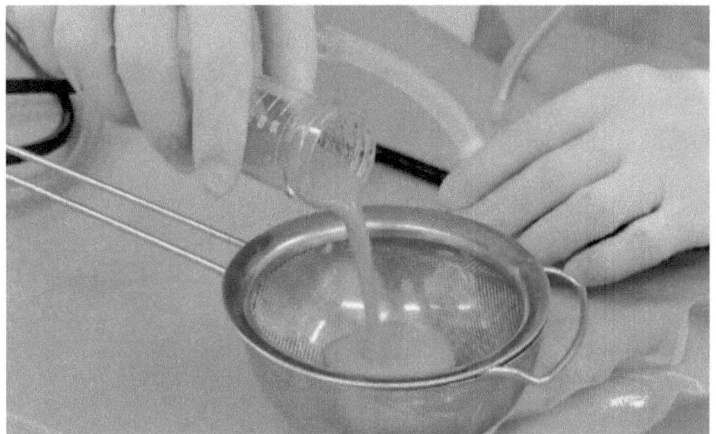

Preparing the fat for injection.

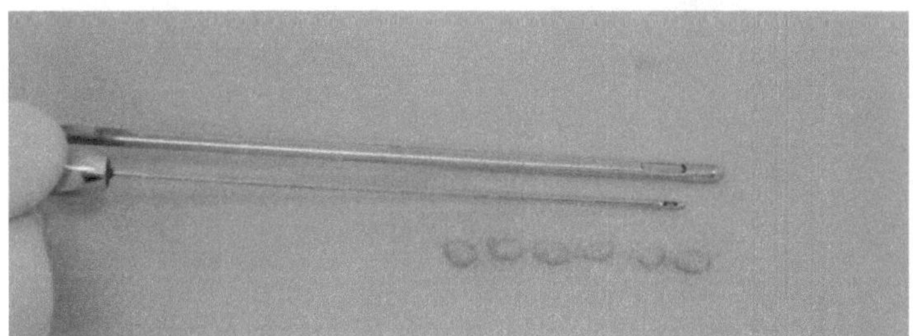

Fat is the best living filler. It contains stem cells that improve skin quality.

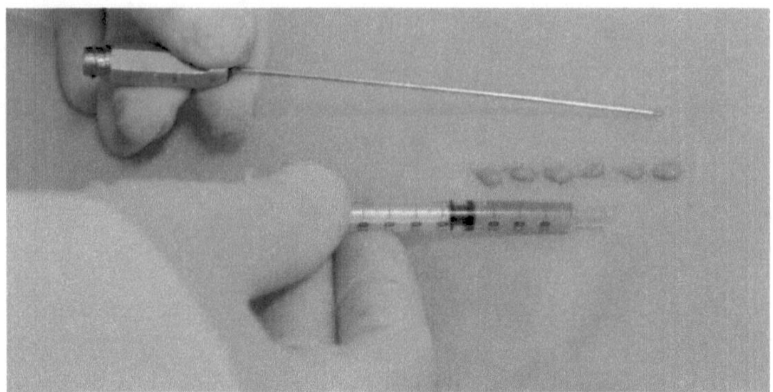

The final product, refined fat cells, ready for injection.

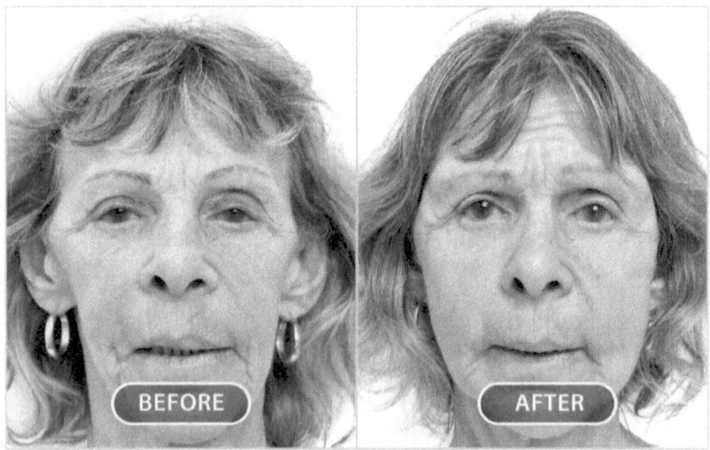

In the before picture, we see a skeletonised face after weight loss. A minimally invasive procedure with fat injections transformed her face. The procedure took one hour. The recovery time was only five days. A neck/face lift would have been the wrong choice for this patient because it would have further skeletonised her face.

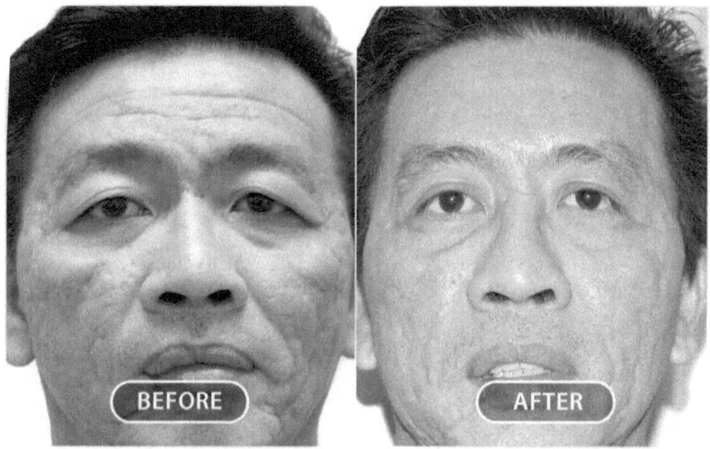

Facial fat injection and upper eyelid surgery. Facelift surgery would have been the wrong choice and cost more.

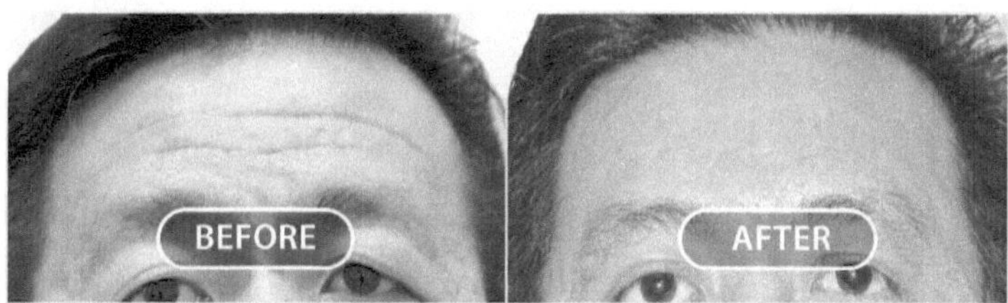

Notice the forehead rejuvenation after fat and stem cell injections. Unlike Botox, it is a permanent result.

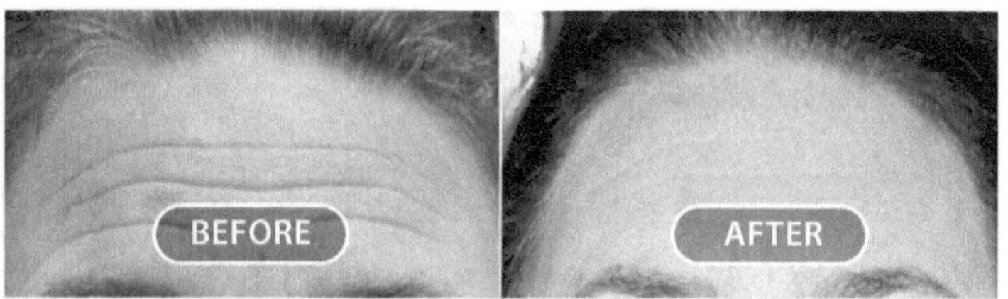

Forehead rejuvenation using fat and stem cell injections is a scarless procedure.

Neck Contouring & Lift

"Don't let your neck reveal your age," said the advertisement on the television. Laura laughed. "Seriously? How is my neck going to reveal my age?"

However, six years later Laura noticed the beginnings of changes in her neck. The skin was beginning to have an aged, crepey appearance, and suddenly her neck muscle bands became visible. She realised with horror, "I have a turkey neck! My neck says I'm 65, but I'm only 50!"

Laura was, at the time, highly resistant to plastic surgery. When she discovered that neck lift surgery is a day-only procedure and can restore the fullness of her neck, she changed her mind.

The result put a big smile on Laura's face. "I don't want to look like I'm 30," she said. "I've earned these lines, and every line on my face tells a story. But that turkey neck was appalling. I am amazed at the result and feel super confident. My neck can keep my age a secret!"

A full and taut neck is one of the signs of youth and beauty. With age, subdermal fullness disappears, and the skin texture gradually deteriorates, leaving behind unsupported, crepey skin. A neck lift, when performed properly, achieves structural support by advancing and tightening the muscles, removing excess skin to restore a more youthful neck.

Neck Liposuction

Necks don't lie about your age. While many women use makeup, Botox and fillers in their faces to look more youthful, forgetting to include their necks in their makeovers only brings attention to the fact that they have had "work" done.

Best-selling author Nora Ephron actually wrote a book in 2006 called *I Feel Bad About My Neck*. Then 65 years old, Nora had resorted to wearing turtlenecks to hide her ageing neck and complained about the lack of a remedy for sagging necks (short of plastic surgery).

The reality is that surgery is the best option even for someone who is sporting a full turkey wattle. A neck-lift performed on its own, or in combination with a facelift, is the best remedy with the most lasting results.

Neck liposuction corrects the dreaded "double chin". The term "double chin" is actually a misnomer. A double chin is essentially a neck problem, not a chin issue. It is due to excess fat in the area of the neck that is directly below the chin, which creates the appearance of an extra chin or double chin.

When this problem of excess fat happens, it does so to varying degrees, with the worst cases appearing like double chins. In less severe cases, the underside of the chin may just look plump without being a double chin. Irrespective of severity, extra neck fat is the source of the problem. As fat is the cause, liposuction is the most sought-after treatment for it.

If the skin is reasonably tight, then liposuction is all that is needed. If the neck skin is very loose, then a neck lift and/or laser may be required, in combination with neck liposuction.

Not all neck fat is extra. It is important, in fact critical, to have a certain amount of neck fat to provide a cushion between the skin and neck muscles. Without it, the neck would look unnatural. Yet, extra neck fat is considered by most to be undesirable. Extra neck fat may be hereditary, and if so, is normally evident in early adulthood. It may also have developed over time; in which case, it is gradual with weight gain. There are also those who have extra neck fat in response to ageing, even in the absence of weight gain. In these cases, fat can accumulate in the neck due to a redistribution of subcutaneous fat that happens with ageing.

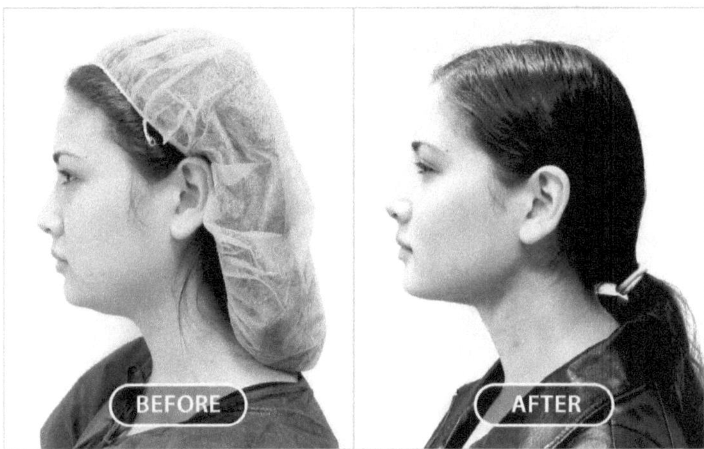

This patient had neck liposuction and buccal fat pads removal.

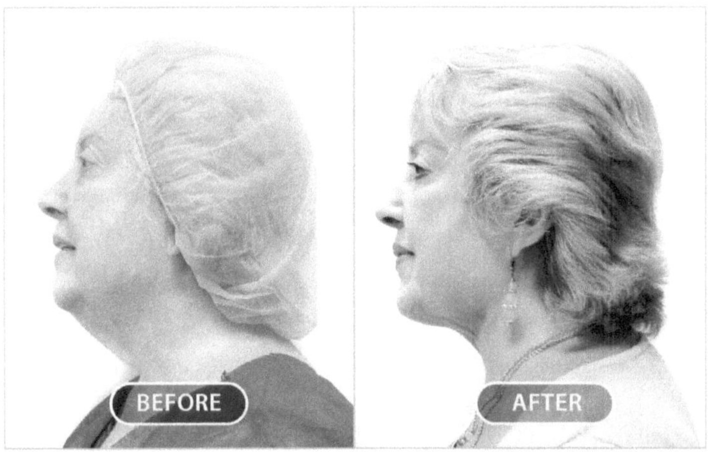

Neck lift and liposuction corrects the dreaded "double chin".

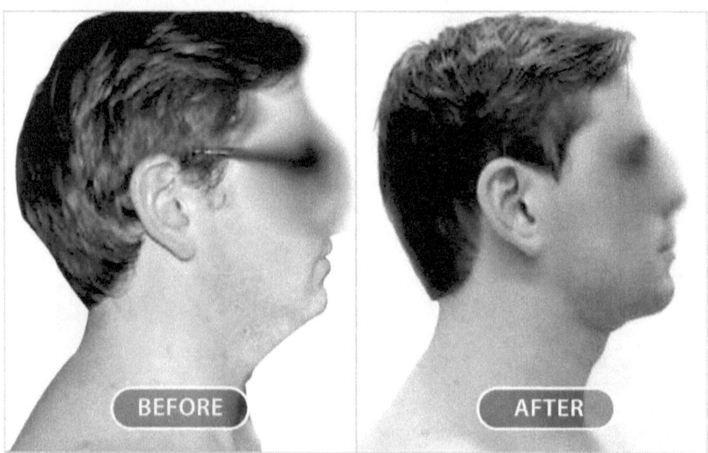

You can see the effect liposuction had on this patient. In the after photo, his chin is more defined, and his turkey wattle is gone, yet his neck looks natural.

Jawline & Jowls Liposuction

"Gramps doesn't have a neck," remarked Jack's four-year-old grandson. While everyone in the room cringed with embarrassment, Jack laughed it off.

Over the years, Jack had put on weight, leading to heavy jowls and neck and back fat that made it look as if he had no neck. His grandson's remark was a wake-up call. His health had been declining due to obesity. Jack realised he might not be around much longer to play with his grandkids and so he went on a strict diet and within two years, had lost half of his excess fat. The trouble was, the extra fat and skin on his jowls did not retreat and he still looked as if he had no neck.

I performed neck liposuction and a neck lift on Jack to create a distinct neck. This gave Jack the confidence to keep going with his weight loss and keep taking charge of his health. Today, at 60, Jack enjoys playing football with his grandsons. He still remembers the day he came home from the surgery, looked into the mirror, and found a well-defined neck that he had not seen for 15 years!

Many who have extra neck fat also suffer the problem of having no distinction between the face and neck. In other words, it is difficult to tell where the face ends and the neck starts. In these cases, liposuction of the neck along the jawline assists to define this area and can be performed at the same time as neck liposuction or neck lift.

Jowls are pockets of fat alongside and above the jawline, about halfway between the ears and the chin. While jowls are typically reflective of loose facial skin (and hence the need for a facelift), liposuction of the jowls can sometimes be completed at the same time as neck liposuction. Provided that the jowls are not associated with markedly loose or hanging skin, liposuction of the jowls can sometimes enable a person to defer a facelift for years.

Neck and jawline liposuction procedures are performed as an outpatient procedure and take 30–60 minutes. I begin by injecting the neck with tumescent fluid, which is a mixture of saline, local anaesthetic and adrenaline, which helps constrict blood vessels, reduce bleeding and prevent bruising. I then make a keyhole incision under the chin to insert the cannula and start drawing out the fat with suction. At the completion of the procedure, the keyhole is closed with fine sutures; this will ensure a virtually undetectable scar under the chin.

Ear Pinning

Luke's childhood was not made any easier by the fact that he had large ears that stuck straight out from his head. His parents didn't allow him to grow his hair, but once he left for university, Luke let his hair and beard grow long to hide his ears. But his ears would still stubbornly peek out, even from his thick wavy hair and bushy beard.

When he graduated, Luke got a job as a town planner. His new job demanded a traditional professional look, which meant the long hair had to go. Luke believed that his protruding ears would make people take him less seriously. At this point, he felt that his career was on the line.

He was very uncomfortable with the idea of plastic surgery at first, but he felt he had no choice. I performed ear pinning surgery to pivot his ears closer to his head because Luke wanted them to stop sticking out. The result was that for the first time, he felt comfortable not hiding his ears behind a mane of long hair. Luke now enjoys his short-haired look and marvels at how low-maintenance it is!

Ear pinning surgery, sometimes called otoplasty, is used to treat a condition where one or both ears are more prominent than usual.

Otoplasty correction works by repositioning prominent ears closer to the head and improving the shape of the ears. Having prominent ears is a relatively common condition which can present in several different ways, including: cup ears, shell ears, bat ears or lop ears. Many patients attempt to conceal unusual or prominent ears under their hair but otoplasty correction is a permanent solution which can help patients feel more confident and allow them to wear their hair any way they like.

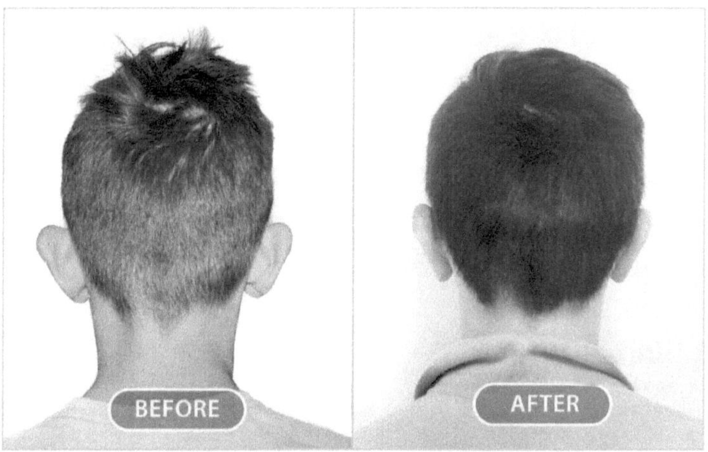

Not only do this patient's ears now lie nicely against his head, but the scars are completely hidden.

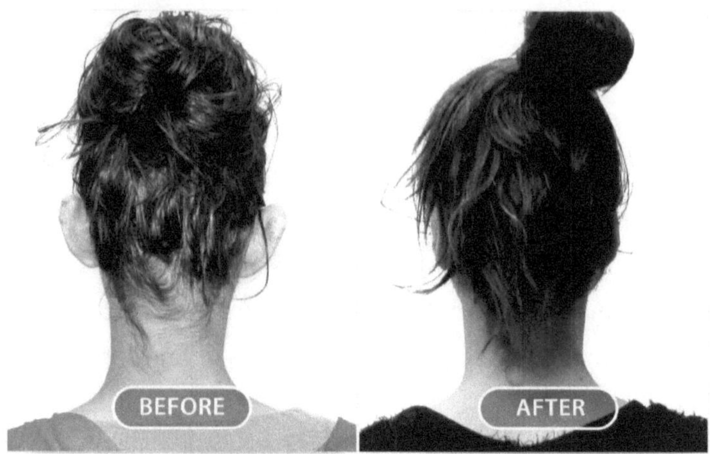

As you can see, the position and symmetry of a patient's ears are important in planning the surgery.

To correct prominent ears or bat ears, an incision is made on the back of the ear to expose the cartilage. Usually, a small portion of the cartilage is removed and then folded towards the head and the ear is stitched back to hold it in its new position. An otoplasty procedure usually takes about 90–120 minutes and the resulting scars are behind the ear where they can't be seen.

Cheek Augmentation

Barbara is one of those beautiful, ageless women. Her face is fairly wrinkle-free, there's a brightness to her eyes, a spring in her step and she doesn't know the meaning of the word "stop". But Barbara has a secret.

Three years ago, Barbara had lost a fair amount of weight, and her face had begun to look sunken. She came to me saying she wasn't ready to look "like an old crone" and asked about her options. We discussed several.

Barbara opted for a soft-touch hyaluronic acid/collagen treatment to restore a more youthful look to her cheeks. This procedure is a simple injection that she currently repeats two-to-three times a year. Barbara loves the natural look of her cheek fillers. Most of all, she loves that she's not using surgery to maintain the fullness in her cheeks.

As we age, cheeks can develop a sunken look that is often made worse by sagging jowls and wrinkles. Cheek augmentation can help achieve a fuller, more youthful look.

There are two options for cheek augmentation (enhancement):

- Soft touch treatment – injectable fillers, hyaluronic acid and/ or collagen is injected with a fine needle. This procedure can be performed in the office with or without the use of a local anaesthetic. It offers instant results that last for about six months. Certain new fillers can have an effect that lasts for up to 18 months. As the effects start to wear off, a top-up injection will be required. I recommend a treatment every three-to-six months for the first year, and then repeat the treatment every six-to-nine months for a year, then once yearly or as needed. This treatment is provided on the day of consultation in the office and may require a local anaesthetic.

- Surgical procedure – By using either the patient's own fatty tissue (biological) or an implant (synthetic), a long-lasting refinement to the areas of the mid-face can be accomplished. This procedure is normally done under general anaesthesia. It takes about 60 minutes and creates a permanent result. For cheek augmentation, using the patient's own fatty tissue, there will be no scar on the face. If implant surgery is chosen, the scar will be 3.5 cm long inside the mouth, with no external scar. The sutures are dissolvable and do not need removal. I recommend fat injections as the gold standard.

Cheek augmentation is often done in conjunction with eyelid fat injections. Fat fillers to the cheek and lower eyelid can restore fullness, soften wrinkles and crow's feet, reduce pore size and lighten lower eyelid darkness. Cheek augmentation with fat grafting produces natural and attractive results which are in proportion to facial aesthetics. This is frequently requested by people who desire more angular and higher cheeks, as well as for people with fat atrophy related to ageing and to minimise the appearance of acne scars. This technique is also useful for concealing obvious silicone implants, minimising the appearance of bulging eyes, as well as correcting facial lipodystrophy and congenital deformities.

The smart surgery is a minimally invasive one that has the most significant impact on the face. It also tends to be the most cost-effective.

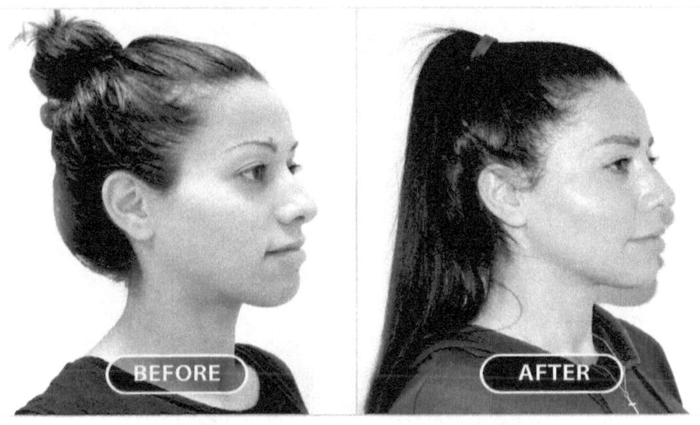

This patient had cheek augmentation surgery.

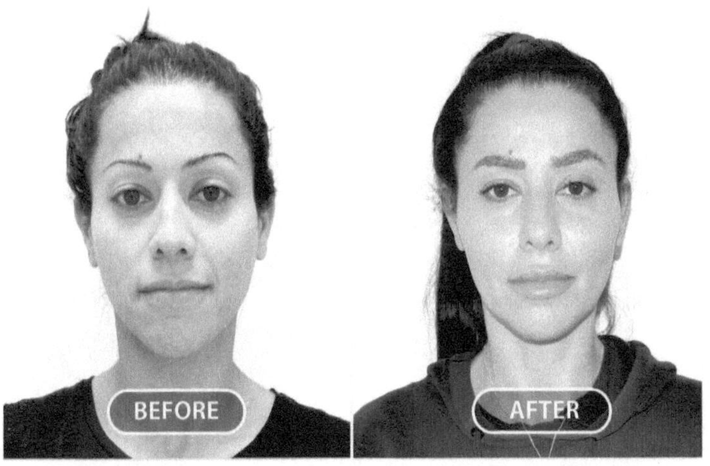

Understanding facial aesthetics is vitally important in producing a natural outcome.

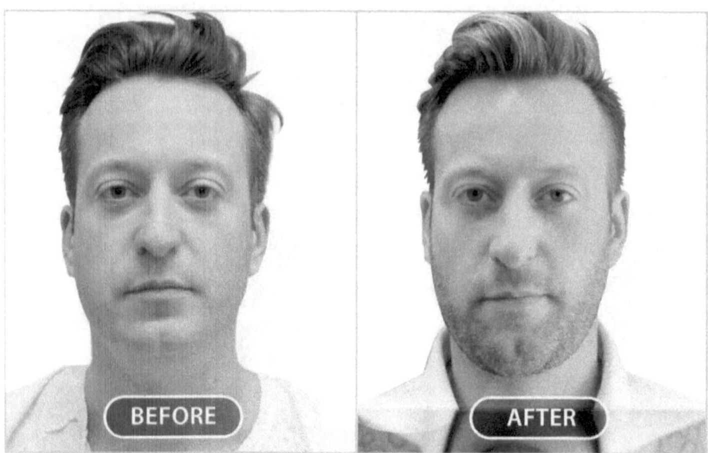

This patient presented requesting rhinoplasty. He was advised that his main issues were lack of volume in the mid-face and chin area, and excess neck fat. I recommended fat injections to augment his cheek and chin area, which I performed together with neck liposuction. The surgery produced harmonious facial features. A rhinoplasty procedure would have been the wrong choice.

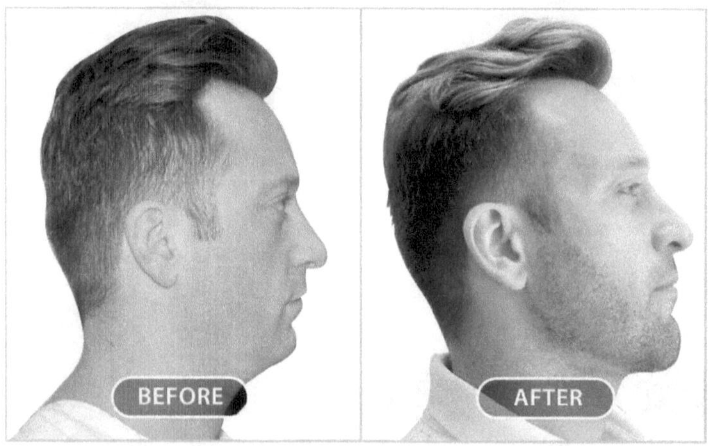

In the after photo, notice the well-defined jaw line and the chin projection.

Chin Enhancement

Bruce always admired the "leading man" look of a strong jawline and chin. Unfortunately, his own chin was weak, which made his nose and forehead appear oversized, as though they belonged to someone else's face. Bruce felt like the dating scene would forever be a string of rejections, as they had in the past. Bruce wanted a dramatic change to give him confidence. His dream called for a surgical procedure to add a chin implant to strengthen his profile.

Only six weeks after the surgery, Bruce was approached by a talent agent who encouraged him to become an actor. Bruce declined. He wasn't interested in being a leading man… he just wanted to look like one. Bruce's dating life, however, took a turn for the better, not only because of his improved appearance, but because of a huge surge in his confidence. Today, Bruce is happily married, with child #2 on the way!

Surgical chin augmentation can have significant effects on the overall facial appearance.

A chin augmentation will strengthen the facial profile by making a weak chin more prominent. This can improve the appearance of the jaw and have a remarkably positive impact on the appearance of the nose and neck area.

A chin augmentation also creates more projection laterally and frontally, resulting in a youthful appearance.

Many types of procedures can be used for chin augmentations, either alone or in conjunction with other operations:

- Soft touch treatment – injectable fillers, hyaluronic acid and/ or collagen are injected with a fine needle. This procedure is done in the office and produces an instant effect that lasts for three-to-12 months. A refined injection technique can achieve a balance between the upper and lower lips, while maintaining the appearance of a natural fullness. After several treatments, the results begin to last longer. This treatment is provided on the day of the consultation in the office.

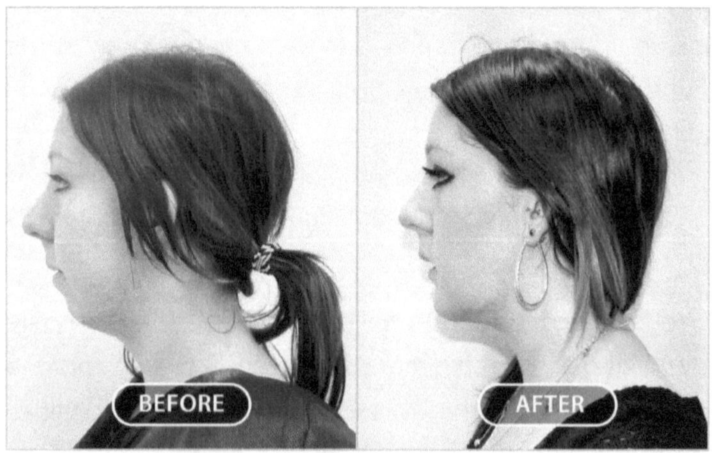

Chin augmentation had a significant effect on this patient's overall facial appearance, even defining her cheeks and neck.

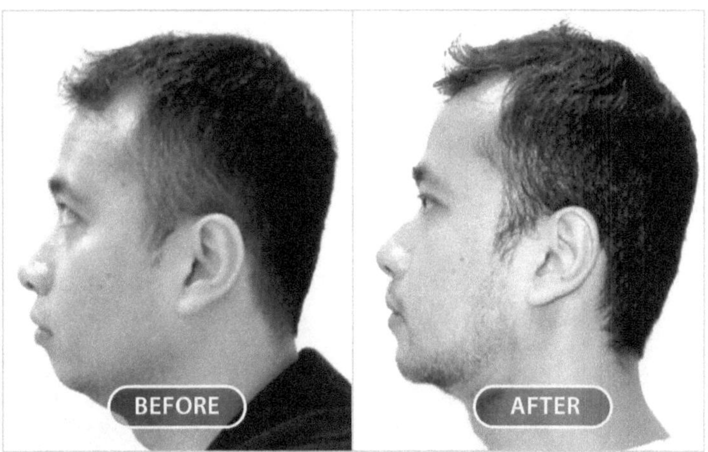

This patient's facial profile was strengthened considerably, and a youthful appearance was obtained.

- Surgical procedure – using either the patient's own fatty tissue or an implant, this procedure creates an attractive, long-lasting refinement to the areas of the lower face and jaw. The procedure is usually performed in a day surgery setting. It takes about 60 minutes and produces a permanent result. For surgical chin augmentation using the patient's own fatty tissue, there will be no scar. If implant surgery is chosen, then the scar will be 3–4 cm long under the chin or unseen inside the mouth. I recommend fat injections for a subtle improvement and a chin implant for a moderate-to-great degree of improvement.

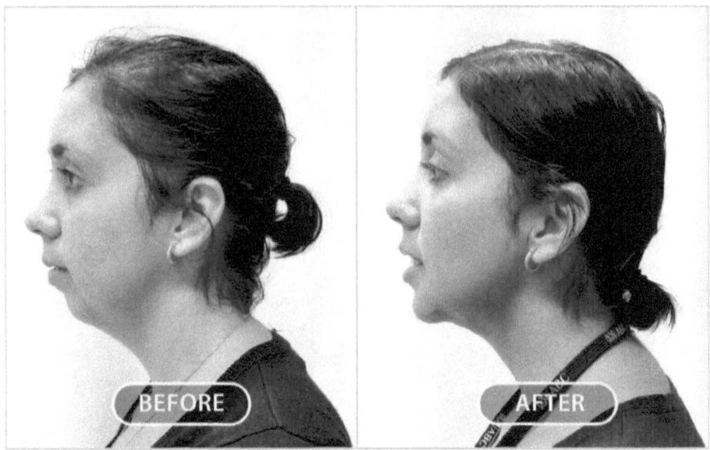

Chin augmentation surgery and neck liposuction.

Lip Augmentation & Lift

When Laurel turned 65, she noticed that her lips had taken on a puckered look. "I look like I've just eaten a lemon!" she exclaimed during our consultation. Laurel had always been proud of her full and sensuous lips. She had no illusions of ever looking like she was 20 again.

"I'm comfortable in my own skin," she said, but the puckered, thin and long upper lip with its downturned corners didn't reflect the happy and vivacious person behind them.

"Even when I smile, my lips don't!" she complained.

Laurel's surgical lip lift, along with fat injections and laser resurfacing gave her a natural look that honoured her age, while restoring her beautiful smile.

As we age, the elasticity of our skin and its supportive elements diminish, resulting in deflated, long and narrow lips with fine lines. The corners get pulled down and create an angry and old appearance.

Lip augmentation, lift and resurfacing produces a natural result when performed together.

There are two main treatment options for the lip:

- Soft treatment (non-surgical) – Such as injectable hyaluronic acid (HA) fillers (including Restylane®, Juvaderm™, Perlane®, Princes®), or natural fat filler, and/or laser to resurface the skin. After a few treatments, the effects may begin to last longer and become more permanent.

  Lip fillers and treatment with HA products are provided on the day of consultation. They usually leave no bruises as they are done from inside the lip.

- Surgical treatment – involves lifting the lip by removing a few millimeters of skin from the top part of the upper lip in what is known as a bullhorn technique. This surgery can be performed in combination with fat injections and laser.

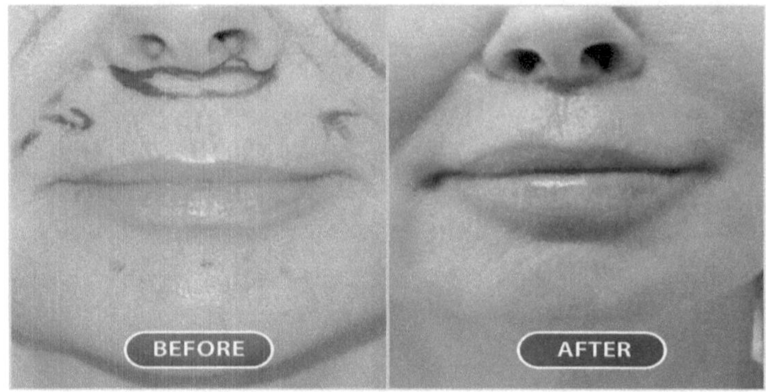

This patient had a lip lift and augmentation.

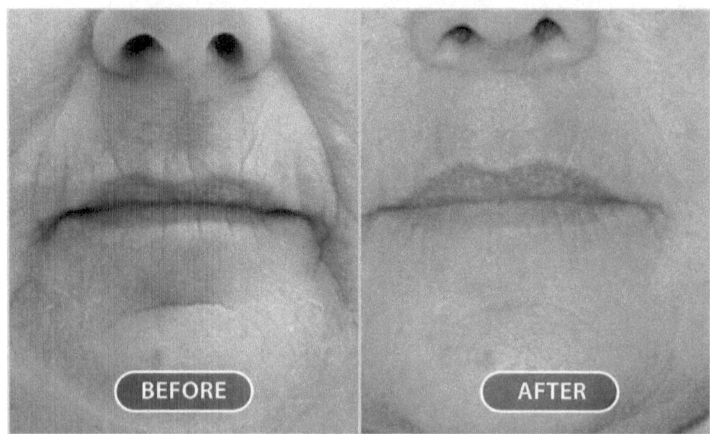

Rejuvenation of the lip and chin area using fat injections, a lip lift and laser treatment.

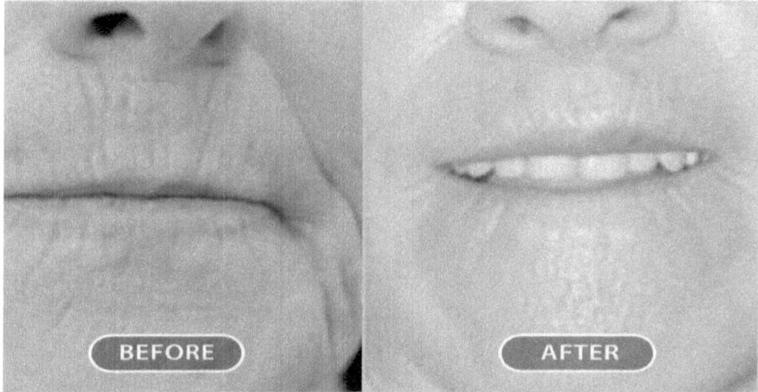

This patient's lip lift and laser treatment resulted in a much smoother and rejuvenated appearance.

Cheek Dimple Creation

Cheek dimples are commonly considered an attractive feature. The procedure for creating cheek dimples is actually quite simple and is usually performed as an outpatient procedure.

This is a surgical procedure that requires the removal of a thin circle of tissue from the inside of the cheek lining. This is done by cutting out a portion of the mucosa (inner cheek skin). This area of missing tissue is then stitched together using quilting and absorbable sutures. The stitch goes through the cheek muscle on one side of the circle of missing tissue, then through the dermis layer of the skin and finally back through the cheek muscle on the other side of the circle. A surgical knot is tied, and a dimple is created.

This procedure can be performed on any kind of cheek; however, the best results are seen when the cheeks are not overly chubby.

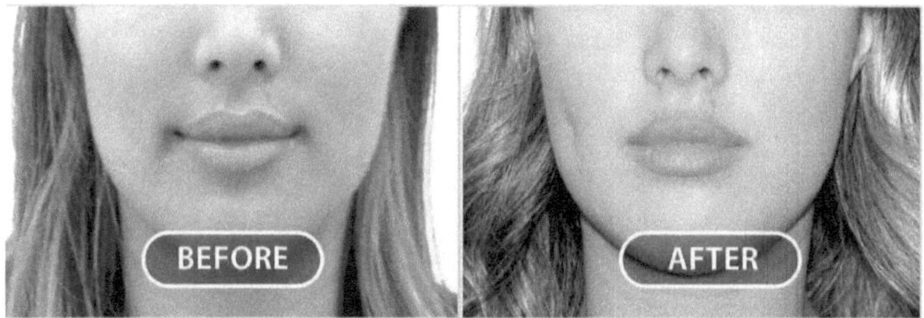

Deep dimple – this dimple shows at rest (above) and at animation (below).

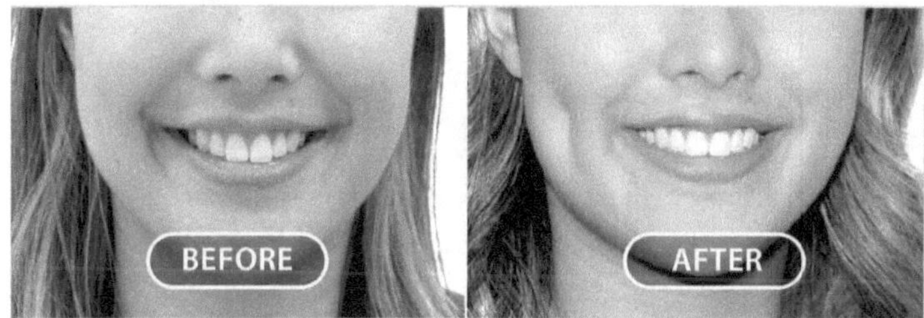

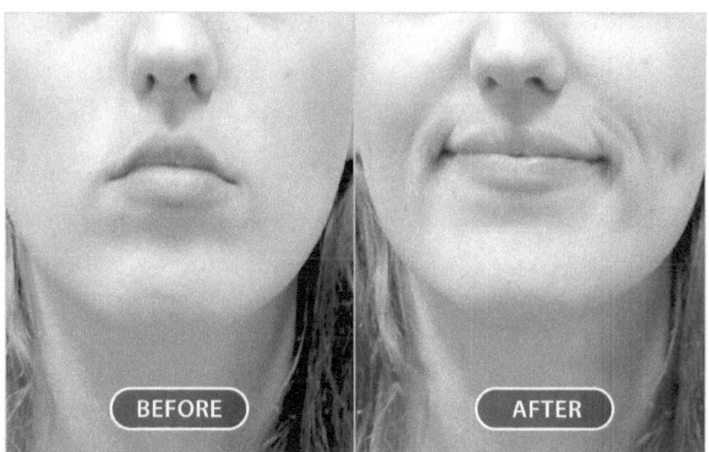

Shallow dimple – the dimple shows only at animation.

Gummy Smile Correction

A gummy smile is a common and unattractive condition defined as the exposure, while an individual is smiling, of more than 3mm of gingival (gum) tissue.

There are a number of surgical procedures that can be used to correct the "gum show" when you smile. The choice of surgical procedure depends on the cause of the gummy smile, which can be due to the soft tissue or bone-teeth malposition.

A simple approach that I use is to transect the depressor septi nasi muscle, at the junction of the nose and upper lip. This will produce a slight drooping or relaxing of the muscles of the upper lip combined with a lengthening of the distance between subnasale and the vermillion border. I routinely combine this procedure with lip filler to increase the vertical height of the wet surface of the lip.

The procedure is often performed in the office under local anaesthesia as an out-patient appointment. There is no visible scaring as it is performed through an internal nasal approach.

Following this minor procedure, the patient will immediately notice a difference in their appearance due to their new smile, which is ready to be enjoyed.

Patients with more complicated cases, or who desire to have additional cosmetic dental work, require different techniques performed by dental specialists called prosthodontists. These techniques include excess gum tissue trimming, a gum lift and/or reshaping of the underlying bones and teeth.

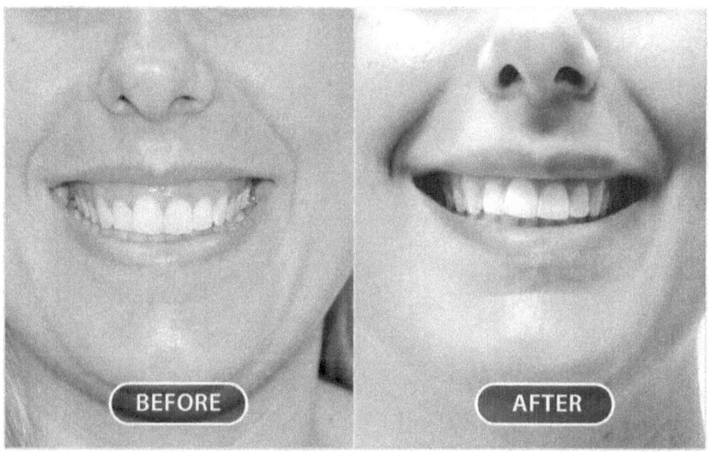

This patient had her gummy smile corrected.

Tracheal Shave Surgery

The Adam's apple is one of the most noticeable gender-related differences between men and women. In men and some women, the small bump known as the Adam's apple may be too obvious because the thyroid cartilage on the throat is large and projects forward.

This projection of thyroid cartilage is not usually noticeable in women and this makes the Adam's apple one of the most prominent features creating a masculine appearance. Some transgender women may also choose to have a tracheal shave procedure, also known as chondrolaryngoplasty, to reduce the size of a prominent Adam's apple as they can feel stigmatised by its presence.

The procedure involves the shaving of the Adam's apple to reduce its size and make the neck and throat appear smoother and less prominent. The key point in this surgery is to avoid damaging the structural support of the vocal cords and to ensure a natural-looking result. I prefer to place the horizontal incision in the neck 2–3 cm higher than the most prominent part of the cartilage, so the scar will be less noticeable and does not adhere to the underlying cartilage and move during speech or swallowing.

The procedure is performed under general anaesthesia as day surgery. Symptoms – including bruising, swelling, a sore throat and difficulty swallowing – can last for up to eight weeks post-surgery. The removal of too little cartilage results in a suboptimal outcome. Alternately, if too much cartilage is removed or the cartilage is removed incorrectly, voice changes such as hoarseness can occur. Damage to the voice is often difficult to correct. Therefore, it is important for tracheal shave surgery to be performed by a skilled surgeon.

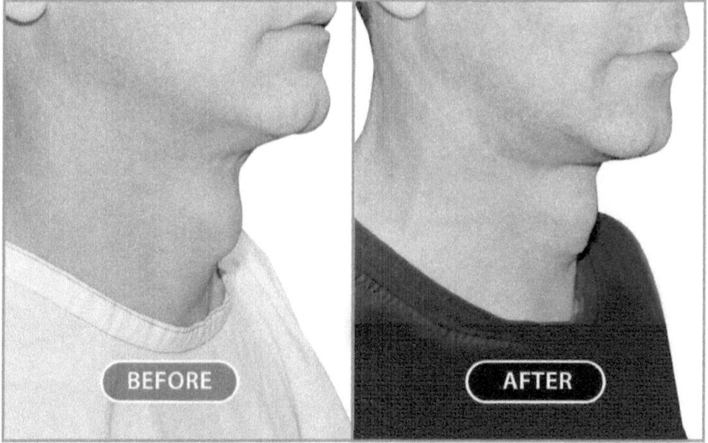

This patient had tracheal shave surgery.

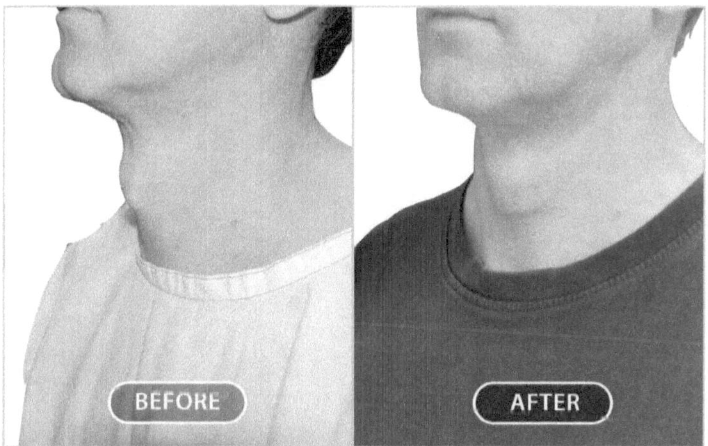

The swelling can last up to eight weeks after tracheal shave surgery.

CHAPTER TWO

Breasts

Breast size and shape are often a big concern for women and can cause serious confidence issues. Breast surgery is one of our most frequently requested plastic surgery procedures because breast changes are common due to developmental reasons, hormonal changes, weight fluctuation, pregnancy or breastfeeding.

Whether you are interested in breast reduction, enlargement, lift, or removal and replacement of an old implant, the best advice is that your breast size and shape have to be in proportion to your body habitus. That means that the width, height and projection of your breasts has to fit within the boundaries of your chest and remain in harmony with the width of your shoulders and hips.

Breast Enlargement

Ever since she was a teen, Janelle was self-conscious about her appearance. Naturally tall and slender, she never developed breasts like other girls her age. Unfortunately, because of her flat-chested appearance, she also suffered teasing from her classmates who would ask her whether she was a woman or a man. When Janelle reached her twenties and it was clear that her breasts would never grow larger, she began exploring the idea of breast enlargement to feel more confident about her body. She chose to have implants done for their superior natural shape and feel. Going up two cup sizes as a result of her breast augmentation meant that Janelle's new look was completely natural for her proportions. Janelle has commented on how confident she feels as a woman. She now enjoys wearing tight clothes where before, she would wear loose clothing to hide her shape and is reportedly enjoying the Sydney dating scene.

Breast enlargement, which is sometimes called breast augmentation, is among the most common procedures I perform. Worldwide, it is one of the most popular procedures for women. Janelle is not alone in her desire for a curvier figure. Studies have shown that more than 50 per cent of women wish to alter the appearance of their breasts. Breast size is a matter of personal choice; however, the modern ideal of female beauty and femininity places an emphasis on breasts that are aesthetically pleasing in all states of dress and undress.

My patients choose to have breast enlargements for five main reasons:

- To increase the size of their breasts;

- Because their breast shape has been compromised by pregnancy or ageing due to inflating-deflating phenomena, fat atrophy or gravitational forces;

- To correct congenital or developmental breast problems which have resulted in smaller breasts;

- Because their breasts are not symmetrical in size and/or shape;

- Because their breasts have been removed as a result of breast cancer; or

- Because of breast injuries, such as scars or burns, that have limited their breast growth.

Deciding to go ahead is a very personal decision which should not be made casually or lightly. I have no hesitation in advising some patients that they do not need the surgery and to save their time, money and effort if I do not feel the surgery is in their best interest. This is especially the case for those women who have good breast volume or are still in their childbearing/breastfeeding years.

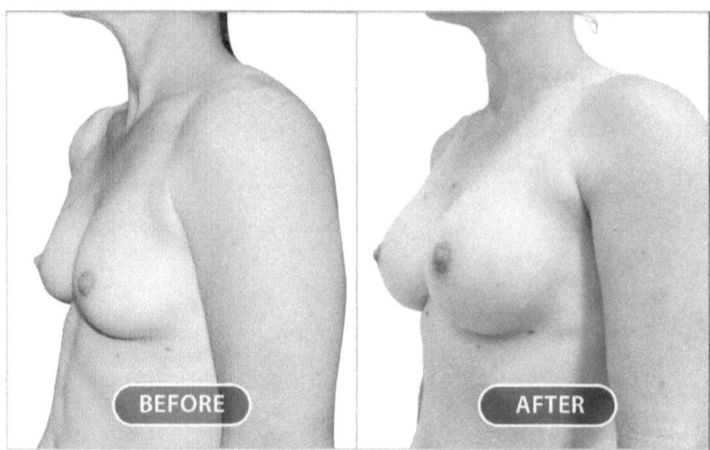

Breast augmentation with 240cc round breast implants. Note the perfect nipple position and proportionate chest.

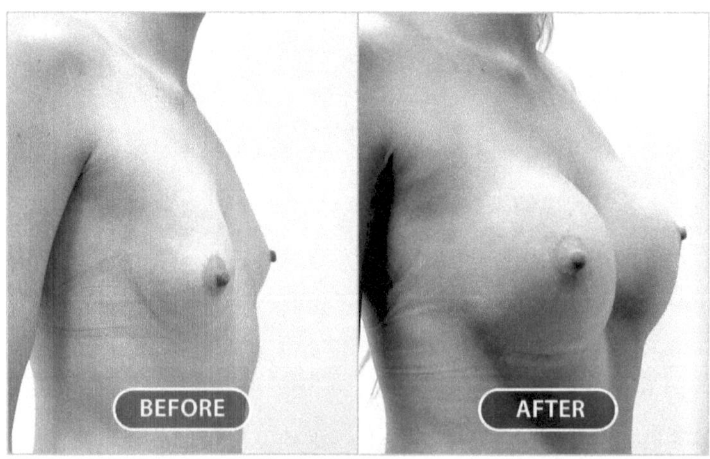

Breast augmentation with 300cc round breast implants. Natural outcome.

Everyone's body is different, and everyone has a different vision of the ideal. There is no one ideal. The shape, texture, profile, width, height and volume of breast augmentation will depend on the patient's body type, desires, and lifestyle. There is no "one size fits all" approach and every woman has her own reasons for considering undergoing breast enlargement.

The surgeon's experience and vision play a significant role in guiding the patient to what is best for them. I do highly recommend to patients that three objectives need to be met with breast surgery: longevity of maintaining perky breasts; aesthetics (appearance) of the breast; and practicality.

It should be remembered that too-large breasts can cause neck/shoulder pain, they will drop quicker and have shorter longevity i.e. the benefits of the procedure will be more short-lived.

Breast enlargement can be achieved through fat injection and/or implant surgery.

Breast enlargement by fat injection is a minimally invasive procedure as it uses fat has been removed by liposuction from other parts of your body. I then purify the fatty cells and inject them into your breasts.

Fat transfer breast enlargement is not new; however, the low survival of the transplanted fat cells has previously been a limiting factor. It has seen a resurgence in recent years due to an improved fat survival technique and the fact that it is a minimally invasive.

It is a great option for women who are looking for a relatively small increase in breast size and would prefer natural results. I routinely use fat transfer when the patient wants her breasts to be enlarged by only one cup size. I also use this technique if the patient has implant rippling, as it is a great way to cover the edges of the implants and enhance the shape.

Another good indication for breast enlargement by fat injection is when patients want to replace their existing implants with larger ones, but their chest anatomy does not allow for a larger prosthesis. Fat injections will give them further enhancement. In those scenarios a single-stage procedure will usually suffice.

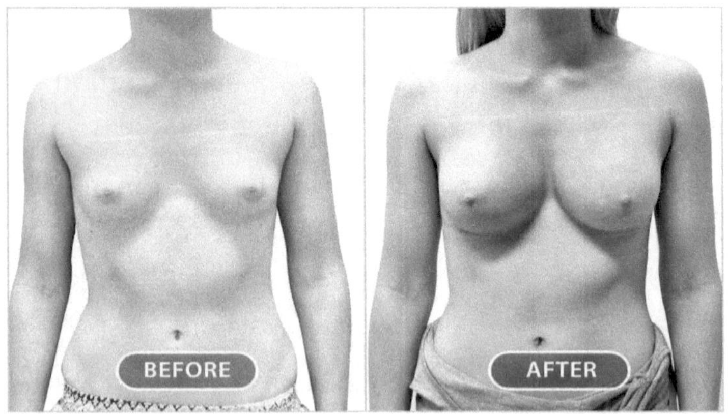

Breast augmentation with 320cc round implants; nice symmetry, upper pole fullness and cleavage.

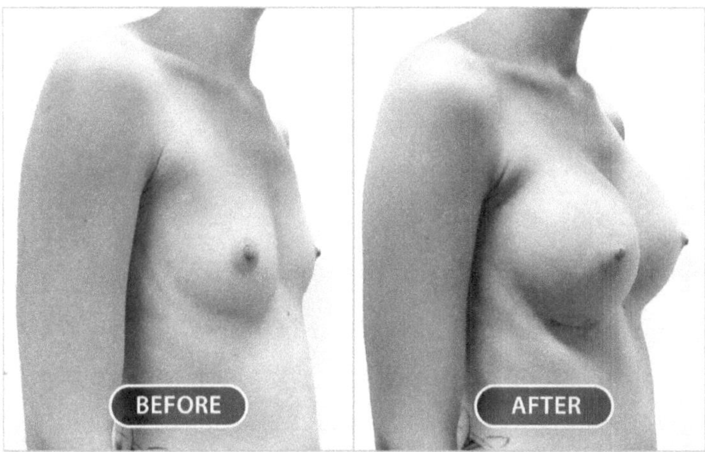

Breast augmentation with 350cc round implants; dual plane.

If the patient wishes to have large increases in her breast size by fat injection, i.e. two-to-three cup sizes bigger, then such an outcome can only be achieved by a multistage procedure. The fat transfer needs to be performed two-to-three times, six months apart as some of the fat that is injected will be absorbed and/or disappear.

The alternative to fat injection is breast enlargement using implants. If the decision to go ahead with implant surgery is reached, then it is vital to choose the right technique, approach and implant.

Silicone implants made in the USA and Europe generally have lifetime guarantees against rupture and/or leakage. Silicone implants are the gold standard. They are made from a rubber shell filled with a highly cohesive silicone gel, which makes them lighter, softer and offers a more natural feel than saline implants.

I avoid using saline implants, due to their propensity for leakage, their unnatural feel and their generally suboptimal results.

Next, we consider the shape of the implants:

- Traditional round breast implants can be either smooth or textured. For under-the-muscle breast enlargements, there is no statistically significant difference between using smooth or textured breast implants. However, for above-muscle breast enlargement, textured round or teardrop implants (see below) are best.

- Teardrop breast implants produce a very natural breast shape and are also known as natural implants or anatomical breast implants. Teardrop implants are made only in coarse texture. The Therapeutic Goods Administration (TGA) in Australia suspended some of these implants in 2019 due to their link with Anaplastic Large Cell Lymphoma (ALCL). This will be discussed in the following section.

Upon making these decisions, the next step is the surgery. It's absolutely vital that the following steps of the "Safe Breast Implants Surgery Technique" are followed by your specialist plastic surgeon to optimise outcomes and minimise complications:

1. The patient is to have a shower the night before or the morning of the surgery.

2. When the patient is under general anaesthetic and before skin preparation with Betadine, I scrub the patient's skin/chest/breast with a Betadine scrub.

3. I then perform routine Betadine preparation and draping.

4. I use intravenous antibiotic prophylaxis 20 minutes before the surgical incision, and two additional doses after surgery and prior to patient's discharge.

5. I use nipple shields to prevent spillage of bacteria into the pocket.

6. I use new instruments in deep planes, that were not used on the skin.

7. I perform a careful dissection.

8. I avoid unnecessary dissection into the breast tissue because this is traumatic and increases patient recovery time.

9. I am careful to maintain haemostasis in order to prevent or stop bleeding.

10. I change my surgical gloves repeatedly as I get underneath the muscle. This will prevent skin contamination deep under the muscle pocket.

11. I use the "No Touch" Technique, as well as another change of gloves prior to handling the implants.

12. I prefer to use a dual-plane pocket, when required.

13. I perform pocket irrigation with correct proven triple antibiotic solution, saline, Betadine or a combination of those solutions.

14. I minimise the length of time during opening, repositioning and replacement of the implant.

15. I prevent friction between the implant and skin, which can contaminate the implant. Friction is avoided by using a protective funnel to guide the implant into the cavity and protect any contact between the skin and the implant.

16. I use a small drain, which is left in place for only 3–4 hours after surgery. It is important that the pocket is absolutely dry prior to the patient going home. The drain will empty the residual fluid/ blood/wash solution from the pocket.

17. I close the cavity in layers, leaving the suture knots away from the implants.

18. I use a closure with deep tissue and dermal eversion technique, especially with the breast crease incision, to ensure minimal scarring.

19. I seal the wound with fine dissolving sutures and do not leave any palpable suture knot directly under the skin surface.

20. I further secure the wound with an additional protective glue barrier.

Such careful execution delivers the best outcomes as well as minimising the post-operative risks and long-term complications.

Such procedures should only be performed by an experienced specialist plastic surgeon. This will ensure the best possible outcome so that the breast augmentation meets the patient's needs, revision surgery is avoided and the procedure doesn't look like an obvious "boob job".

An excellent breast augmentation looks natural, with a gentle sloping off the chest wall to natural fullness, natural cleavage without webbing between the breasts, and a certain amount of perkiness. It lasts for about ten years without long-term issues such as rippling, neck pain, double bubble or bottoming out.

Breast augmentation is a 60–90 minute procedure that, when performed correctly, can dramatically alter the way a woman feels about her body.

For women who want to maintain their current size or have larger breasts volume and currently experience sagginess in their breast tissue, breast augmentation can be performed at the same time as breast lift surgery.

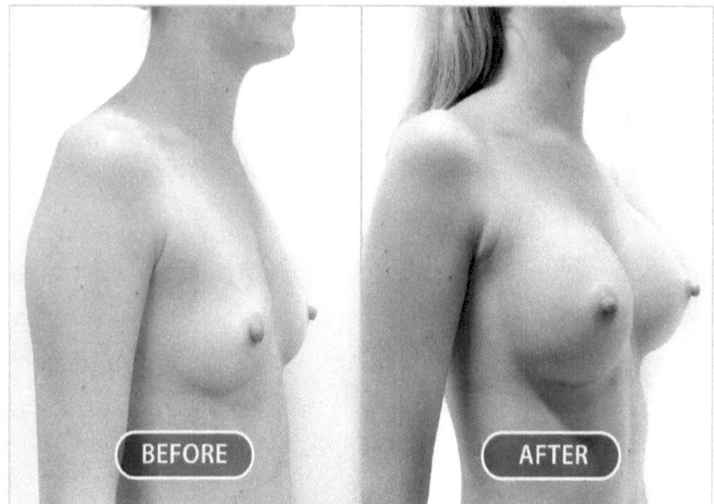

Breast augmentation with 360cc round breast implants; dual plane.

Breast Implant Removal & Replacement Surgery

Breast implant removal surgery is performed under general anaesthesia and takes approximately two hours. It is usually performed as day surgery.

The three most common breast implant removal surgery techniques include:

1. Breast implant removal with capsulectomy – incisions will be made in the same place as the breast implant surgery was performed. A part or full section of the capsule surrounding the implants will be removed and sent for histopathological examination.

2. Breast implant removal and replacement with capsulectomy – as above with insertion of a new set of implants. Usually patients request higher projecting and slightly larger implants.

3. Breast implant removal with breast lift – some patients require a breast lift when they have their breast implants removed or replaced with smaller ones. The surgery is designed to remove the excess breast skin and tighten the breast tissue to provide better support. The areolas are often re-sized to better fit the new shape of the woman's breasts.

Whilst recovery from breast implant surgery varies from person to person, it is usually smoother than the initial breast implant surgery. However, if you have a breast lift after your breast implants have been removed, your breasts will feel tight for a few weeks.

Most women are able to return to work five days after surgery and experience minimal discomfort. If you've had breast implants removed due to capsular contracture, there will be more discomfort and the recovery time will be longer.

Breast implant removal scars typically heal very well and are often inconspicuous. It is important to note they heal in stages with the process taking three-to-four months.

You will need to avoid lifting anything over five kilograms or exercising excessively for the first six weeks after your surgery. While you will usually be able to resume normal activity after six weeks, your breasts will take three-to-six months to settle into their new position.

When a highly trained and experienced plastic surgeon performs breast implant removal/replacement surgery, the complications and risks will be minimal. However, it is important to note that the risks and complications can include:

1. Blood collection or what is known as haematoma;

2. Infection, which may necessitate the removal of the implants;

3. Development of thick, red and painful scars, which may last for a few years;

4. Numbness of the breast and/or nipples; and

5. Breast deformity or sagging of the breast area.

Breast implant removal surgery can address a variety of concerns, including: capsular contracture, implant malfunction and dissatisfaction with breast size. If a woman chooses not to replace the breast implants, a breast lift may be required to address the skin that has been stretched.

With breast implant surgery, a revision or replacement surgery is usually required within 10–15 years.

In some cases, breast implant removal and/or replacement procedures need to be performed in two stages. The first stage is the removal of the implants and capsulectomy. The second stage is the insertion of new implants and/or breast lift.

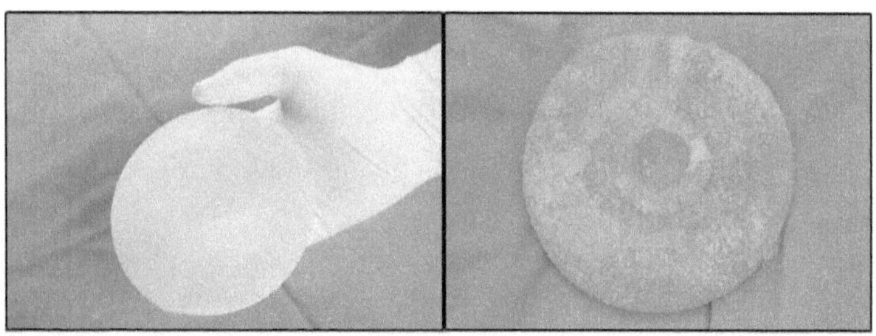

New breast implant   Explanted old implant

Breast Implants Associated Anaplastic Large Cell Lymphoma (BIA-ACL)

This is a rare and highly treatable type of lymphoma that can develop around breast implants. BIA-ALCL occurs most frequently in patients who have breast implants with highly textured surfaces. This is a cancer of the immune system, not a type of breast cancer. When caught early, BIA-ALCL is usually fully curable by removing the implants and the capsule. It takes an average of seven-to-ten years after implant insertion before the lymphoma develops.

The most typical presentation is a fluid swelling around the breast implant and in the space between the implant and breast implant capsule.

The Australian Therapeutic Goods Association (TGA) announced in 2019 it is considering regulatory action regarding breast implants. This included suspending and recalling certain types of breast implants following an extensive review of an apparent association between Anaplastic Large Cell Lymphoma and some implants.

Anyone with breast implants needs to ensure they have their implants checked regularly by their specialist plastic surgeon.

While the majority of the implants are safe, and many women live full and rewarding lives with implants, the impact of Breast Implant Associated Anaplastic Large Cell Lymphoma (BIA-ALCL) is noticeable.

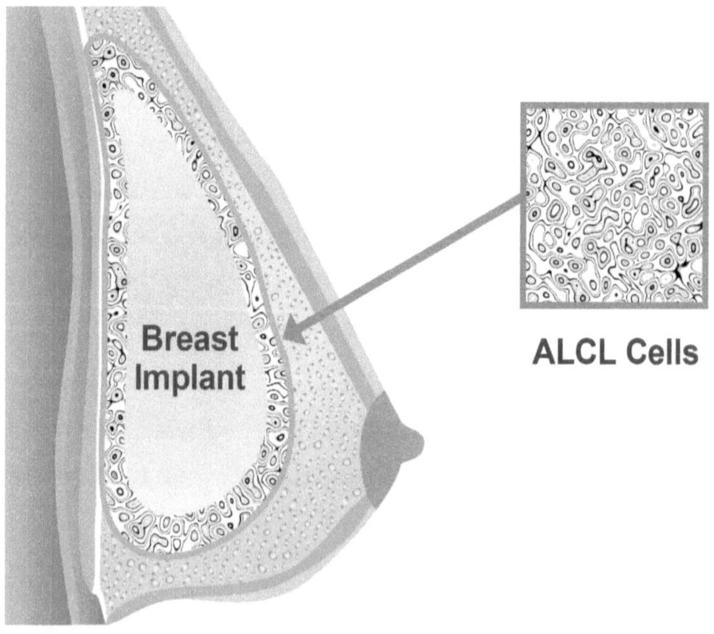

There are around 35 million women (60 million implants) in the world with textured breast implants. As of January 4, 2021 (ABDR, 2021), there were over 900 confirmed cases of Breast Implants Associated Anaplastic Large Cell Lymphoma (BIA-ALCL) worldwide and 123 cases in Australia. There have been over 32 deaths from late diagnosis of the disease worldwide, including four in Australia (Lonescu et al, 2021[1]). Estimates of risk and incidence have increased significantly recently, reaching 1 in 2,969 women with breast implants, and 1 in 355 patients with textured implants after breast reconstruction, based upon current confirmed cases and implant sales data over the past two decades. The incidence of BIA-ALCL cases in Australia is higher than expected, based on the population. About 1 in 7 of all cases reported globally are Australian cases.

1. Lonescue P. et al. New Data on the Epidemiology of Breast Implant-Associated Anaplastic Large Cell Lymphoma. *European Journal of Breast Health* 2021 (Oct); 17(4): 302–307.

However, it is important to put things into perspective by stating that the incidence of breast cancer among women who do not have breast implants is one in eight. Therefore, the incidence of BIA-ALCL is considered to be rare.

A unifying theory has been proposed by the authors of a paper in an epidemiology journal. The authors believe that the four factors likely to cause BIA-ALCL are:

1. Use of textured implants (with a higher risk for high surface area textured implants);

2. Bacterial contamination at the time of surgery to reach a threshold to cause inflammation;

3. A patient's genetic predisposition. The incidence of BIA-ALCL is lower in Asian populations;

4. Time for the process to develop, which is usually a seven-ten year incubation period.

I recommend following strict protocols to minimise bacterial contamination. See the 20 points under the heading, "Safe Breast Implants Surgery Technique", earlier in this chapter.

These 20 points include: scrubbing the skin with Betadine; the use of a protective sleeve or delivery system; intravenous (IV) antibiotics; changing gloves frequently; the use of "No Touch" techniques; washing the pocket with saline; minimising the time of exposure; the use of techniques to minimise tissue injuries; careful haemostasis (to avoid bleeding); layered closure; and careful atraumatic dissection to reduce the risk of devascularised tissue.

I am proud to report that our clinics in Sydney have never had a reported case of Breast Implants Associated Anaplastic Large Cell Lymphoma.

Breast Lift

Natalie always felt inferior about her sagging breasts. A mother of three children, Natalie noticed that after breastfeeding each child, her breasts would sag just a little more each time. Being a relatively small C cup to begin with, Natalie became extremely self-conscious that her breasts had not only deflated but were now (in her words) "heading toward the floor". Because of her insecurity about her small, deflated breasts, she started to avoid intimate relations with her husband Ben, unless she could keep her bra on or make love in total darkness so he could not see her breasts. As this soon began affecting her relationship with Ben, Natalie decided to take charge and see me for a breast lift consult.

The breast lift, or mastopexy, is one of my most frequently requested plastic surgery procedures. Breast droop is common due to weight fluctuation, hormonal changes, pregnancy or breastfeeding. Other women desire a breast lift because they wish to improve on their natural breast shape.

Breast droop following pregnancy can be caused by a hormonal softening of the ligaments that hold the breasts up and by tissue stretching. Changes in breast size during pregnancy and after pregnancy can sometimes be quite dramatic. This is often accompanied by a loss of breast tissue, which means the breasts appear to sag and the upper half of the breast looks flat. Minor degrees of breast droop can be effectively corrected by breast augmentation alone but, if the nipple is at or below the level of the breast crease, a breast lift will be required to recreate youthful looking breasts with high nipples.

A breast lift is often combined with breast augmentation if an increase in breast tissue is also required to restore the breasts to their former fullness, shape and position. Many patients who complain of breast sagginess, or breast ptosis as it is known in medical terms, will respond well to a surgical lifting of the breast tissue known as a breast lift or mastopexy.

Natural-looking breasts are the ultimate goal of breast enhancement surgery. This can be achieved through careful planning, a comprehensive breast examination and analysis. This includes precise breast measurements and a detailed discussion with the patient. An implant trial will be performed to decide on the size of the breast implants. Breast augmentation can be performed by fat injection using the patient's own fatty tissue or with breast implants.

The breast lift procedure creates a fine scar on top of the areola only (mini-lift), or a lollipop scar around the areola and vertically down (short scar breast lift) or a lollipop and a horizontal component in the breast crease (inverted T, a full breast lift).

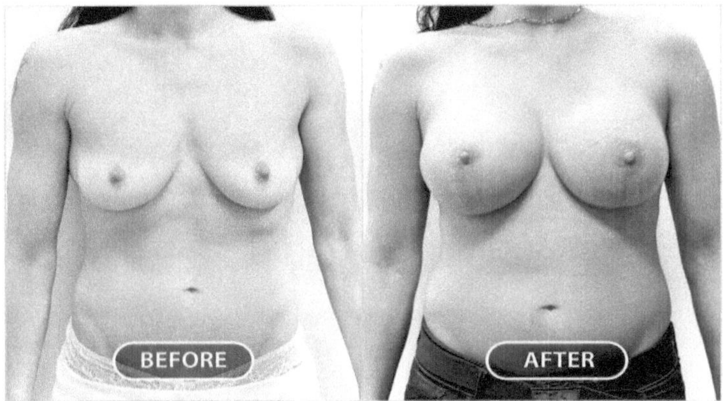

Breast lift and augmentation surgery. Note the sharp cleavage and proportionate breasts.

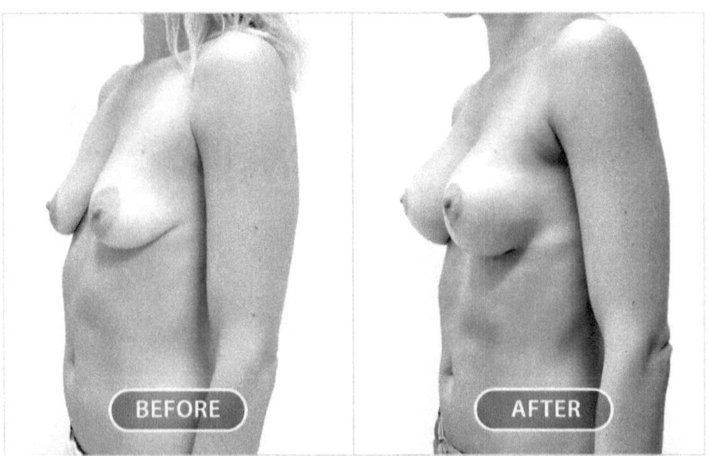

Natural breast lift and augmentation outcome using 260cc round, silicone implants. The patient's areolae were reduced and the nipples lifted.

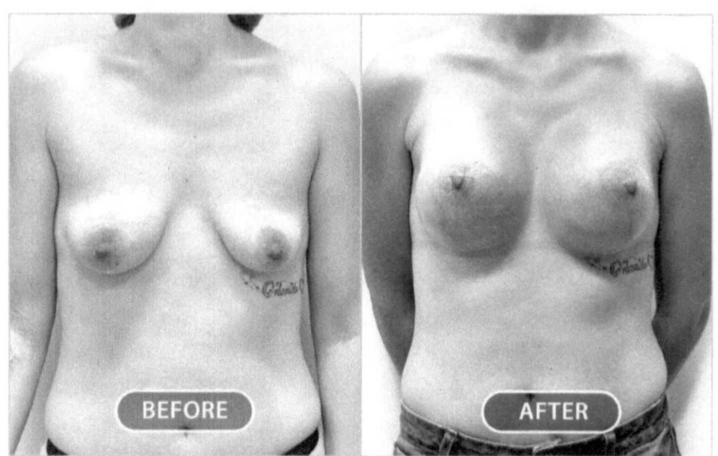

Many women choose to have a breast lift due to breast droop, caused by weight fluctuation, hormonal changes, pregnancy or breastfeeding.

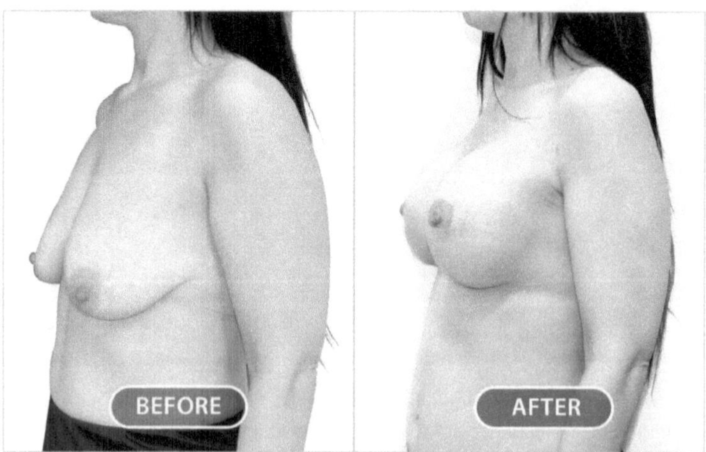

Breast lift and augmentation surgery using 375cc round, highly cohesive implants. This included repositioning of the nipples.

Breast Reduction

A big-chested girl since she was 12, Jill felt weighed down by her breasts. She enjoyed playing tennis and volleyball but always had to wear two compression bras just to keep "the girls" in check. "Jill's hills", as she called them, eventually caused the formation of deep grooves on her shoulders from the weight of the breast tissue supported only by narrow bra straps.

After giving birth to two children, her breasts grew even larger. After she lost her baby weight, however, Jill's breasts seemed even more disproportionate to her hips and belly. Not only had they also begun to sag, but she developed lower back problems from the weight of her breast tissue.

Every time she looked in the mirror, Jill felt matronly and unattractive, which was exactly the opposite of how she wanted to feel as a 30-year-old mum. Jill decided to have a breast reduction done.

Jill had 1.8 kg of breast tissue removed, which gave her immediate relief. The tissue was sent for histological examination in a laboratory and was reported to be free of any abnormal cells.

Lateral chest liposuction was also performed to further define the outer border of her breasts and make her more comfortable.

The lift and reduction surgery produced a healthier, lighter and happier Jill.

Breast reduction surgery is normally performed under general anesthesia as a day surgery or as an overnight stay. The procedure takes two-to-four hours to perform, depending on the size of the breasts and the amount of reduction required. It is a very satisfying procedure for patients as it improves their posture, takes the pressure off their neck and shoulders, and gives them better quality of life.

Note: For discussion of Male Breast Reduction ("man boobs") see **Chapter 6: Plastic Surgery for Men**.

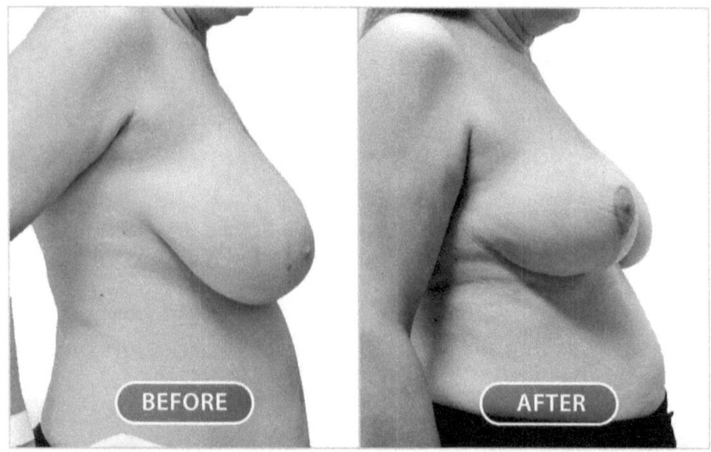

During this woman's breast reduction surgery, approximately 650 grams of breast tissue was removed from each breast, and she is now two cups sizes smaller. Her quality of life was greatly improved as her back pain diminished.

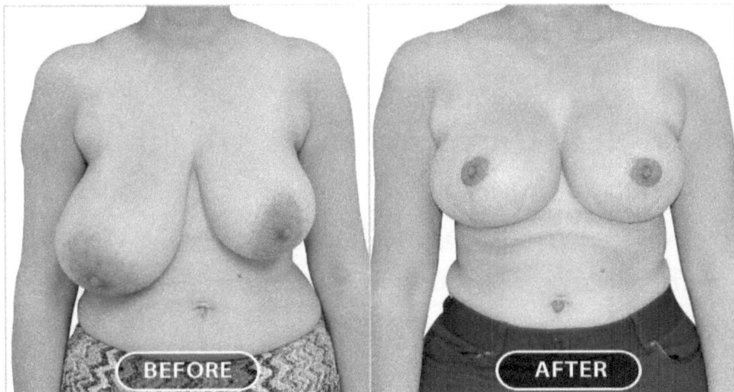

When a patient has to deal with a large breast size and disproportion, the body must constantly compensate, which overtaxes muscles in the shoulders and back, causing prolonged or increasing pain.

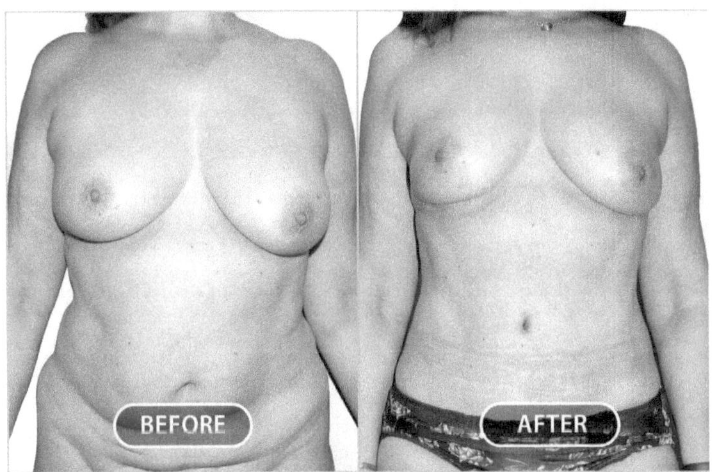

This patient underwent a tummy tuck and breast reduction by liposuction.

Areola Reduction

Areolas are the pigmented part of the breast skin. When areolas appear disproportionately large due to genetics, pregnancy or heavy breasts, they can be resized and reshaped with an areola reduction procedure. A wide areola diameter can be reduced to suit the rest of the breast tissue/nipple size and shape. This 45–60 minute procedure is usually performed as day surgery. It can be performed alone or in combination with breast augmentation or breast lift surgery.

Inverted Nipples Correction

Helena hated undressing in the locker room after swimming practice. She was self-conscious about her inverted nipples (even though she loved the ability to go braless without the "headlights"). She felt that her inverted nipples were unattractive and childlike, and so even in her sexual relations, she would refuse to go topless unless the lights were dimmed. When Helena discovered that inverted nipples could be fixed through a simple surgical procedure, she jumped at the chance. Today, she enjoys new confidence as well as increased sexual enjoyment.

This one-hour procedure is done under local anaesthesia, which makes the nipple area numb. I perform a keyhole surgery that leaves no scarring and minimises downtime.

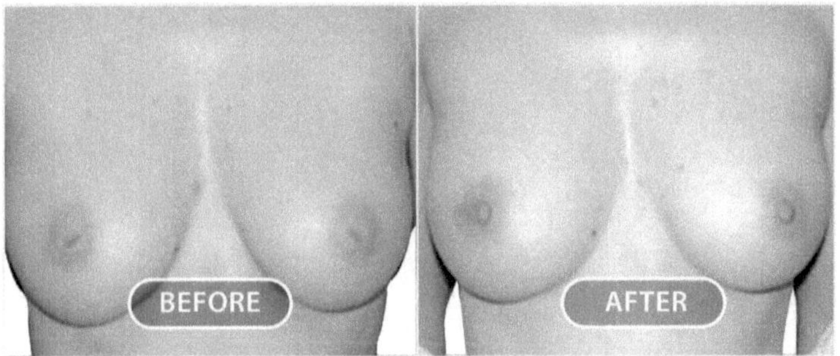

An inverted nipple repair may be done for several reasons.

Nipple Reduction

Nipples that are large (due to genetics or breastfeeding) can be resized and reshaped, making them appear more natural and less aged. Nipple reduction can be performed alone or in combination with breast augmentation or breast lift. The 20-minute procedure is completed through keyhole surgery and leaves virtually no scars.

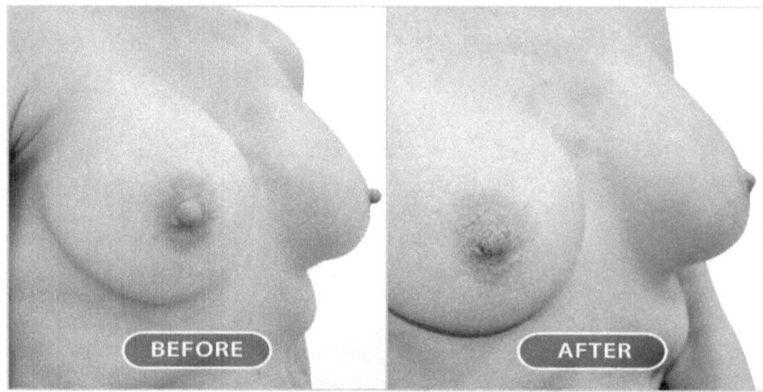

Before and after nipple reduction.

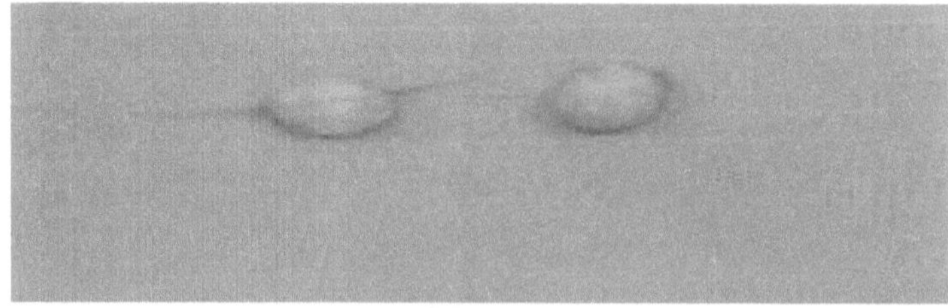

Amputated nipples

Abdomen and Body

Extra skin, fat and weak muscles around the abdomen can be caused naturally by pregnancy, old age or even stress-related weight gain that proves resistant to an improved diet and exercise.

As we age, fat is often redistributed to our hips and abdomen. Known as "stubborn fat areas", these may be hard to shift through exercise and diet alone.

How we feel about our bodies can have a huge impact on our general wellbeing. For example, disliking our own body can have a negative impact on our relationships with other people. Many patients opt for a tummy tuck, which is sometimes called abdominoplasty, because they want to wear a wider variety of clothing and improve their personal body image.

Tummy Tuck & Body Lift

For most of her adult life, Colleen had been fighting with a stubborn tummy bulge that wouldn't go away. Two pregnancies (including a C-section as a first-time mum), a stressful divorce and then the onset of menopause left Colleen struggling with stubborn excess fat around her belly that refused to respond to diet or exercise. Colleen worked with a personal trainer, but nothing seemed to flatten her belly, so she looked into what was involved with a tummy tuck.

She discovered that the procedure produces a long scar; however, since it would deliver the outcome that she was wanting, Colleen immediately started to be interested in the surgery. The procedure allowed her to finally attain a flat, sexy belly, flat mons pubis and an hourglass figure.

Colleen has no regrets about her choice, but says, "If you'd asked me in the first few days after surgery, I would have had a different opinion". Colleen was warned to expect up to seven days of recovery and found it difficult to walk for three days post-surgery.

"I am so pleased now especially since this surgery, when done properly, is once in a lifetime. I did this surgery for myself, not for my husband or anybody else. I wanted to look hot, and there's no shame in that. I don't have to cover up my belly anymore. I'm still young and want to look good for as long as possible!"

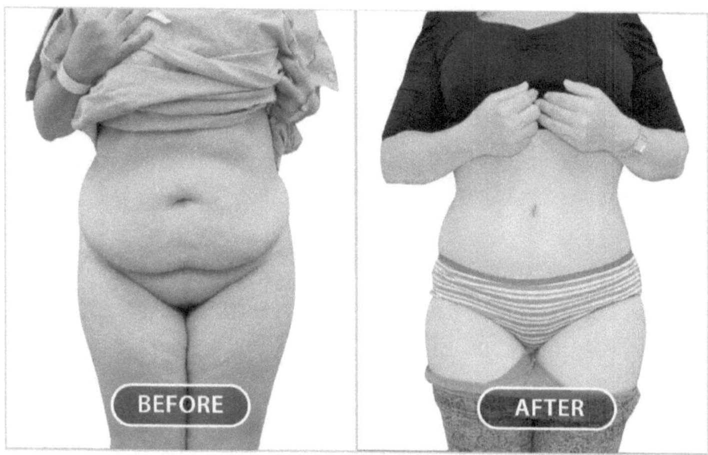

You can see the amazing transformation in these patients after their tummy tucks and liposculpture.

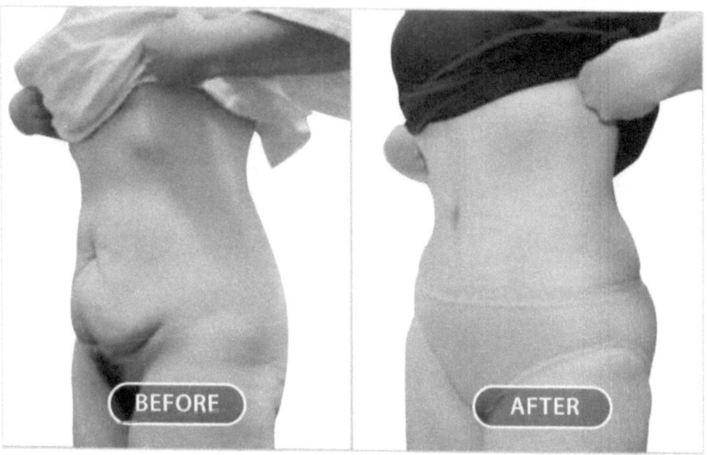

Notice the creative upper tummy abs shadow line.

Tummy tuck, or abdominoplasty, is a surgical procedure which removes excess skin and fat from the middle and lower abdomen and tightens the abdominal muscle wall and connective tissues to create a firmer, flatter abdomen and slimmer waist.

It has become one of our most commonly requested plastic surgery procedures. To get the best possible results, I routinely include liposuction as a complementary procedure to abdominoplasty to recontour and reshape the entire abdomen, flank, waist and any "love handles".

I often perform a body lift in conjunction with abdominoplasty. This procedure achieves the reduction of excess tissue around the hips and back. The body lift is a significant operation used for total body lift and contouring. It involves longer recovery times and must be approached with special consideration for patient safety.

During the procedure, I make a long incision across the abdomen, running from one hip bone to the other and within the pubic area. This is normally done so that the future scar will be covered by swimwear or underwear. If required, a second-round incision is then created around the umbilicus (tummy button), to free the navel from its surrounding tissue.

Next, I will separate the skin from the abdominal wall right up to the ribcage and pull back the resulting flap to show the vertical muscles in the abdomen. These muscles will be tightened by drawing them in together and stitching them into position. The skin flap is then stretched back down, and the excess skin is removed.

The procedure takes about three hours and requires a two-to-four-day hospital stay. If a patient is suitable for a mini-abdominoplasty or mini tummy tuck, the skin is separated only as far as the navel rather than up to the ribcage, the incision is much shorter, and it may not even be necessary to move the navel at all. The patient may be able to go home on the day of surgery.

The tummy tuck scar will vary depending on the tightness of the closure and the patient's natural healing abilities. I pay exceptional attention to place the scar as low as possible in the pubic area, so it is hidden under clothing. I also implement techniques to minimise scaring, such as progressive tension and SFS (superficial fascial system) techniques. For most patients, the scar looks like a fine white line, once fully healed.

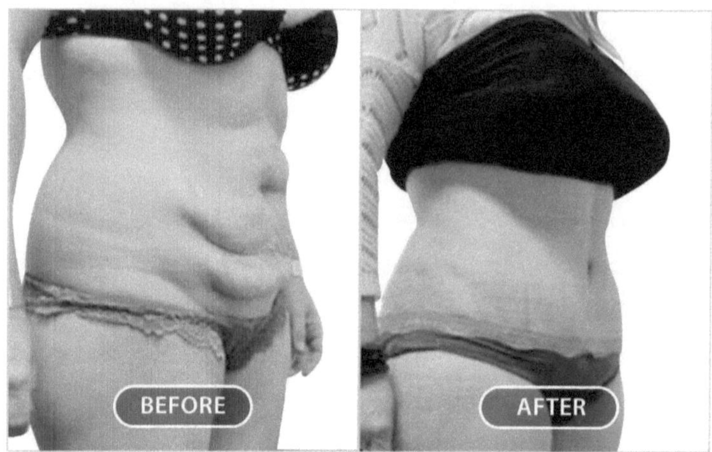

Notice the new small belly button, the waistline liposuction, the low-seated scar and the attractive midline groove.

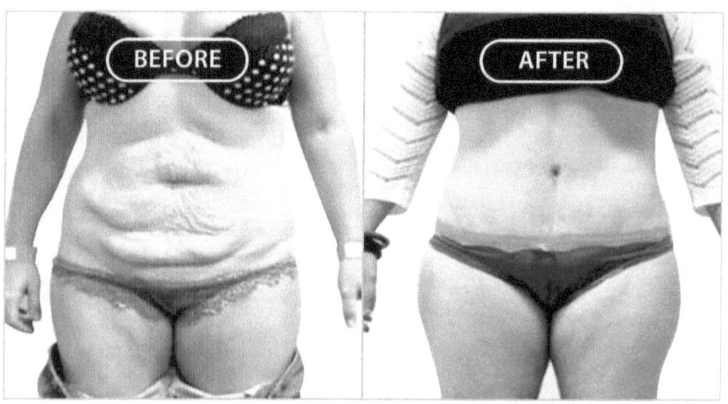

Notice that the scar is completely hidden by the patient's clothing.

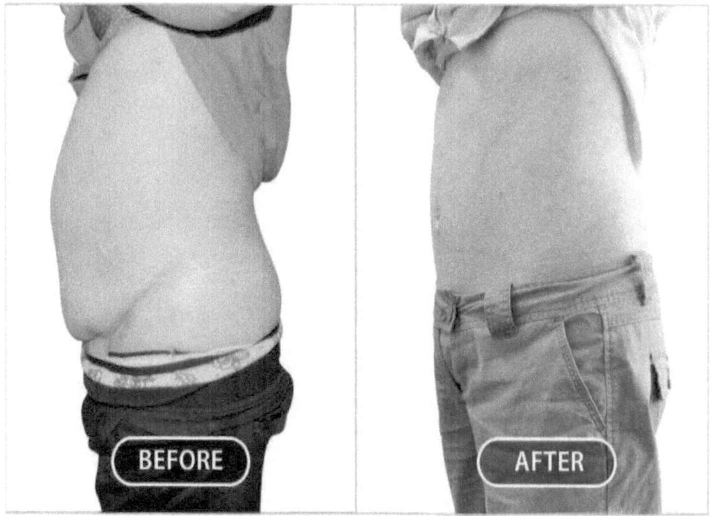

This patient had a tummy tuck and liposculpture.

Liposuction

Fiona had grown up in a family of overweight people. All her life, she was told that "it runs in the family" and that people were powerless to take charge of their weight. This didn't sit right with Fiona, who was starting to gain weight in all the wrong places. "What about exercise?" she would argue. "What about diets?"

Each question was answered, "Well, you can do a little, but in the end, it's in your genes."

One day as Fiona was trying to fit into her favourite dress – and failing – she'd had enough. "NO," she thought to herself, "there is no way I'm going to end up looking like my mum, my sister or my aunt. I'm only 23, and I look like a toad!" But at the same time, the thought of going to the gym was intimidating.

Liposuction removed several kilograms of fat from around Fiona's belly, love handles, buttocks, thighs and upper arms. She completely transformed her body in one day, which inspired her to join a dance class and weight training class. Today, Fiona is a passionate advocate of fitness. Liposuction gave her the "jump-start" and confidence she needed to join the gym. Fiona is studying to become a certified nutritionist and fitness coach, and best of all, she is inspiring her sister to take charge of her weight!

Liposuction is a procedure to remove unwanted fat deposits from specific areas of the body, which are resistant to exercise and diet. The body areas that can be sculpted include the: abdomen, waist, arms, thighs, face, neck, back, buttocks, hips, knees and ankles. It is a powerful procedure for altering body proportions. To achieve the best results, careful planning with a clear outline of the overall goals is essential.

The traditional liposuction technique is rarely used these days. Most plastic surgeons now use either power assisted liposuction (Microaire) or ultrasound liposuction (also know as Vaser).

Liposuction can take between 30 minutes and three hours, depending on the complexity of the case. During the liposuction procedure, the unwanted fat is first liquefied by injections of saline solution combined with local anaesthetic and a vasoconstrictor, which restricts local blood flow. I then make a tiny incision and introduce a hollow, stainless steel tube called a cannula into the deep fat layer. Working on this layer is safer than working on the superficial layer as there is less risk of injuring the skin. I push and pull the tube through the fat layer. As the cannula moves, it breaks up the fat cells, which are sucked out with a vacuum pump or syringe.

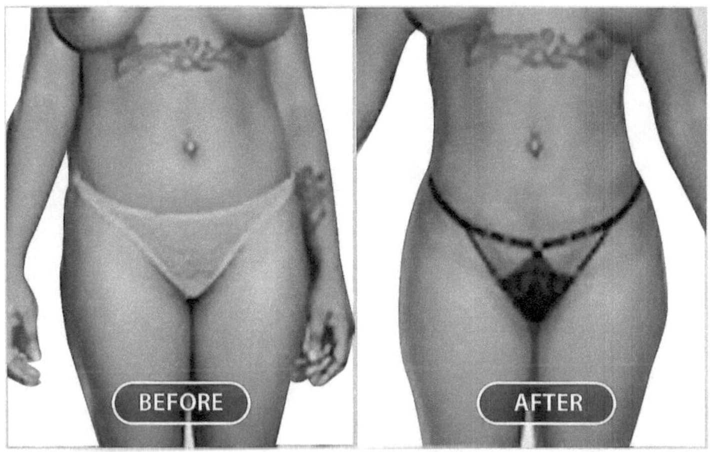

Liposuction can be focused on areas of need to obtain specified results. Notice the skin shrinkage after artistic liposculpture.

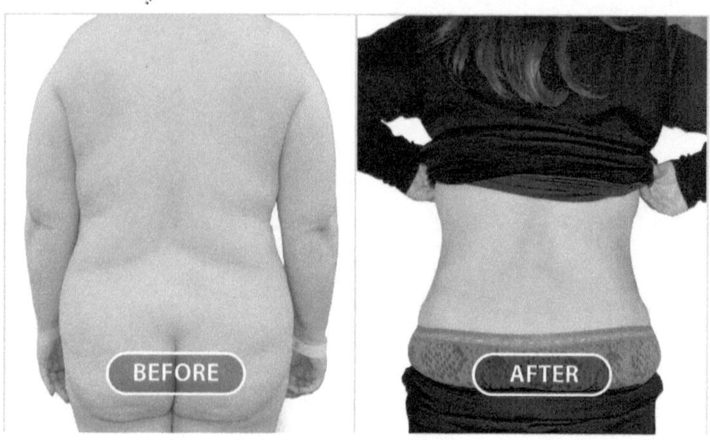

These patients saw powerful results to the abdomen, waist area, back, hips, buttocks and thighs post liposculpture.

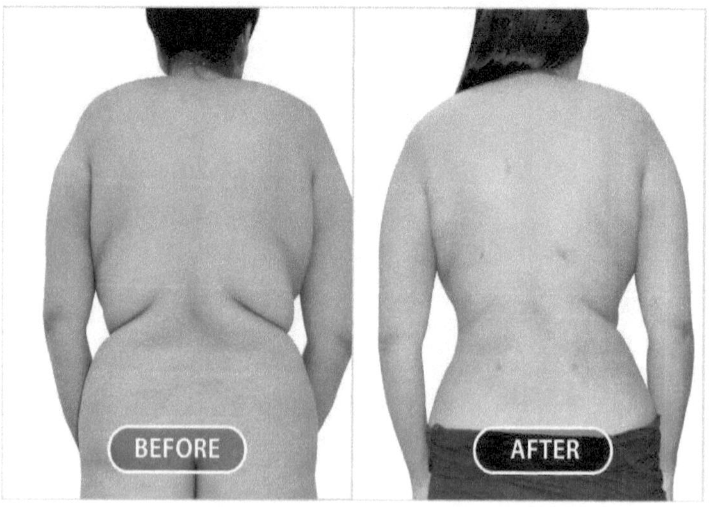

Posterior recontouring by liposculpture.

Post Weight Loss Plastic Surgery

Dania says, "After my gastric bypass, it took me two years to schedule an appointment to have a body lift done. After I lost 54 kilograms, I had this huge gut, which at that point was a blob of skin. Nobody admits to having work done, so I didn't know that it was even a thing to have all this extra stretchy skin removed. The reality is, people think that when you lose weight, you're set. They're wrong. If you have skin that's hanging off you, it's like you're trying to wear a bodysuit that's six sizes too big, so of course, you're not going to feel great about yourself. When I found out about a body lift that would finish my weight loss transformation, I knew it was stupid to wait any more. I had a tummy tuck, butt lift and overall tightening of the skin on my arms and legs. Did it work? Oh yeah. Today I get nothing but compliments and look like I'm in the right size body. Sexy!"

Many people who lose a significant amount of weight end up with excess skin that won't shrink back to its old dimensions. Others feel that certain body parts have succumbed to gravity and that they are slowly sliding to the floor. Where a facelift can give the impression of youth, it is only a partial remedy if other parts of your body tell a different story. Body makeovers are a "complete package" that restore a youthful look everywhere it's needed or desired.

Individuals who are overweight due to genetics, habits or post-pregnancy, are willing to try anything to lose weight and get back into shape. A small percentage of them can achieve their goals through diet and exercise. An even higher percentage of people, however, find that their weight interferes with exercise and confounds the problem. They find themselves in a "Catch 22" situation; they can't exercise because of their weight, and they are unable to lose weight because they can't exercise.

One popular solution for individuals caught in this situation is to have bariatric surgery. This surgery is performed by a bariatric surgeon and is designed to modify the stomach and intestines so that weight loss is possible. Bariatric surgery has been very effective in producing significant weight loss for many people who feel they have no other option.

Plastic surgery procedures following massive weight loss are generally extremely gratifying for both the patient and the surgeon. The outcomes are usually dramatic and offer a significant functional and aesthetic benefit to the patient.

These procedures address the loose skin that remains after the weight is gone. While someone is overweight, the skin stretches to accommodate the increased volume of fat. After weight loss, the skin often fails to tighten, and therefore it sags or even hangs. It acts as a continuous unattractive reminder of your previous weight and figure.

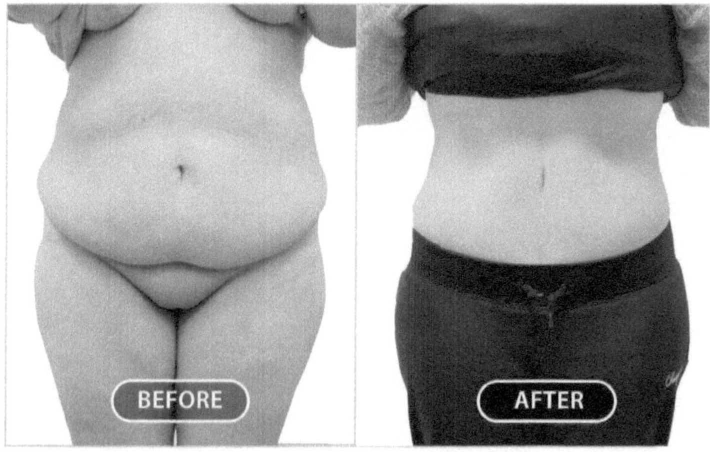

Excess skin removal is often necessary after excessive weight loss. A number of procedures were performed on this patient, including pubic lift, repaired muscle separation, and liposculpture.

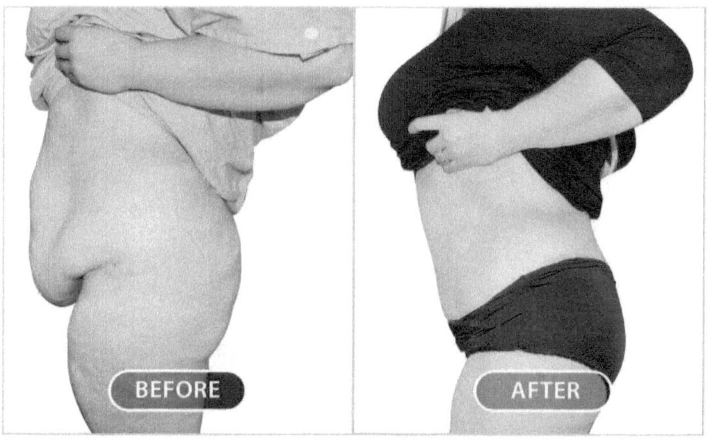

Post weight loss abdominoplasty.

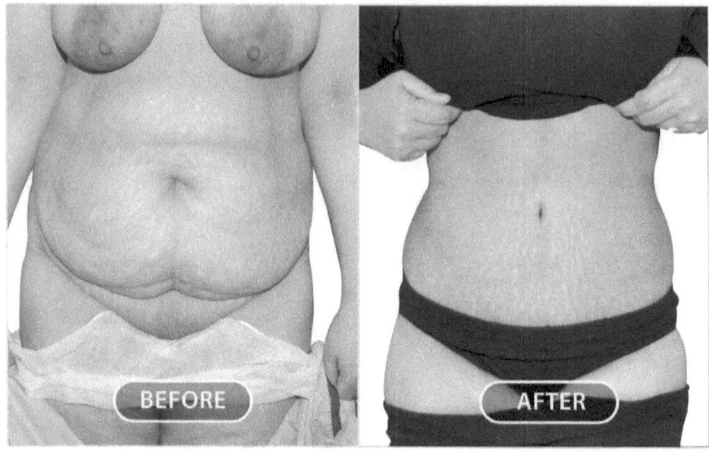

Extended radical abdominoplasty, liposculpture, pubic lift and umbilical reshaping.

Unfortunately, diet and exercise will not tighten the skin (exercise never tightens skin, only muscles). The only way to tighten and/or remove loose skin is through surgery.

Depending on an individual's unique situation, there are several surgical options:

- A facelift to eliminate loose face and neck skin;

- A tummy tuck to eliminate loose abdominal skin;

- A pubic lift to eliminate the overhanging part of the mons pubis;

- An arm lift to eliminate loose arm skin;

- A breast lift to eliminate loose breast skin;

- An inner thigh lift to eliminate loose inner thigh skin; and

- A buttock lift to eliminate loose thigh and buttock skin.

Most individuals who achieve significant weight loss often require a few of the above operations. The surgery is tailored to fit the patient's needs, beginning with the area of highest concern. Most substantial weight loss patients prefer to start with a tummy tuck and breast lift, with or without breast enlargement, for shape enhancement.

The body lift is performed under general anaesthetic in a hospital and takes five-to-seven hours depending on its complexity. It must not be entered into lightly. As with any surgery, there will be scarring. The more skin that requires removal, the longer the scar. For a body lift, scars will range from along the lower abdomen, around the hips, and toward the buttock crease.

There is an additional scar in each groin crease due to the inner thigh lift. One way to look at it is that this operation exchanges one cosmetic problem (loose skin) for another (scars). Generally, those with very loose saggy skin following substantial weight loss are likely to find that this trade-off is worthwhile. Those with only a small amount of looseness will perhaps decide they do not want the scars.

Stretch Mark Removal

After two pregnancies, Carrie had developed deep purple stretch marks all around her belly. She didn't wear her stretch marks like a "badge of honour" simply because none of her friends with children had such awful and prominent purple stretch marks that year after year, refused to fade. Carrie avoided going to the beach unless she was wearing shorts and a t-shirt. Try as she might with creams and lasers, which promised to eliminate her stretch marks, nothing worked. After consulting with me, I assured her that her stretch marks could be removed and she could once again enjoy the smooth skin she had before she had children.

Carrie says, "I have never before had such confidence about my post-baby belly. I dress differently. Recently I bought my first bikini since I was 17! I'm proud of how I look."

Stretch marks occur during phases of rapid weight gain. The skin stretches to accommodate increased body volume, and it will tolerate significant stretching over a short period of time (such as throughout pregnancy). At some point, however, skin reaches a threshold, and the deepest layer will tear instead of stretching further. After this tearing happens, the overlying skin remains intact but looks thin and streaky. These streaks are known as stretch marks. Unfortunately stretch marks are permanent.

Some people opt for laser removal of stretch marks, and there are physicians who claim that lasers are effective in removing stretch marks. However, there is no evidence to support this. Most plastic surgeons think that lasers are ineffective in treating this problem.

Lasers are effective in removing, vaporising and breaking down tissues. They do not usually repair tissues. Stretch marks signify torn tissue; therefore, improvement should not be expected from laser treatment. Furthermore, clinical studies have shown no improvement after laser treatment. The only real improvement comes by using a surgical procedure.

Abdominal stretch marks occur mainly below the belly button. The only way to eliminate stretch marks is with a tummy tuck. During a tummy tuck, much of the skin below the belly button is removed. Therefore, stretch marks in this area are also removed. There is no other proven treatment to remove stretch marks.

Mummy Makeover

*"After four kids, what did I expect my body to look like,"
said Kim, "Angelina Jolie?"*

*Although she joked about it, Kim was extremely
unhappy with her post-baby body. And yet, she didn't
go ahead with plastic surgery because she felt guilty. "I
couldn't spend money on just me, on vanity. I was afraid
that I would be laid up for a while, which is not really an
option when you've got four little ones running amok."*

*Kim had a change of heart, though, when she noticed
that her friend Elisabeth, a mum of two, had "suddenly"
lost a lot of weight and looked ten years younger. Kim
asked Elisabeth what she had done.*

*Elisabeth looked sheepish for a moment, but then
she lifted her chin and proudly said, "I had a mummy
makeover. I decided to put myself first for once. I realised
that if I was unhappy, everybody was unhappy. I decided
to be a role model and teach my kids that it's okay to put
yourself first sometimes."*

*Kim thought deeply about what her friend had said.
She remembered Elisabeth wearing baggy clothes to hide
her body, and the change in her friend was remarkable.
Elisabeth really did look 20 years younger. Her waist was
slim, her breasts were perky and her radiant smile was back!*

*Kim consulted with her husband about the financial
implications of the work she wanted to have done. To*

her surprise, he supported her. "This is really important to you, isn't it?" he asked. When she meekly said yes, he replied, "You deserve it. You're a fantastic mum, you're the love of my life, you work so hard to take care of our family and why shouldn't you be happy? You sacrificed your body to be a mum, but it's not something you have to live with if you don't want to."

Today, Kim looks and feels like she did before she became a mother. She says, "There's one thing that Elisabeth said that struck a chord – that it's okay to put yourself first sometimes. Mums often don't, and then everybody's miserable because of it."

Although having children is one of life's greatest gifts, pregnancy, childbirth and breastfeeding can take a huge, and often irreversible toll on a woman's body. It leaves many mothers frustrated and dissatisfied with their appearance.

With our fun-loving beach culture, Australian mothers are usually keen to maintain their figures and body confidence. But after having a baby, some body parts will never return to their original shape or condition, no matter how much weight they lose or how much toning they do.

A mummy makeover is a combination of plastic surgery procedures, which are custom designed for each woman to achieve the desired results.

The procedure is popular with women in their twenties, thirties and forties; in particular for women who've finished having babies and want to reclaim their body.

The Mummy Makeover includes some or all of the following plastic surgery procedures:

- Tummy tuck (also known as abdominoplasty);

- Pubic lift and mons pubis reduction;

- Liposuction to the tummy, hips, flanks and thighs;

- Breast enlargement, breast lift (with or without implants) or breast reduction; and

- Vaginal rejuvenation, including labiaplasty and/ or vaginoplasty.

Labiaplasty is a procedure that involves trimming the excess inner vaginal lips. Vaginoplasty is performed to narrow and restore the vaginal muscle to pre-childbirth status. Vaginoplasty helps prevent uterine prolapse, increases friction during intercourse, as well as restoring sexual confidence and pleasure.

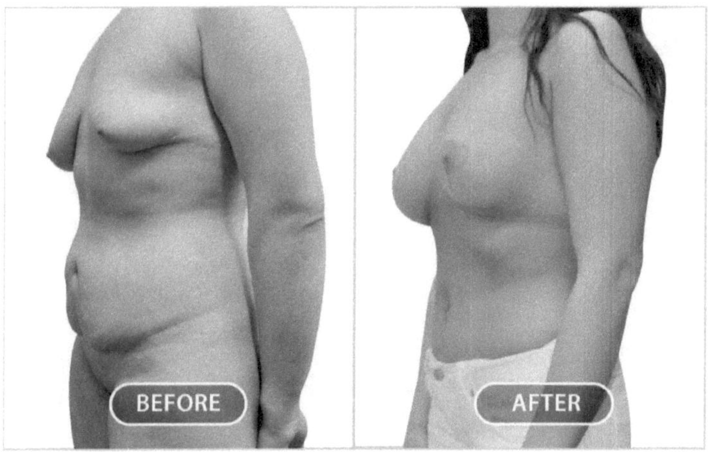

Mummy makeover: tummy tuck, liposuction and breast surgery.

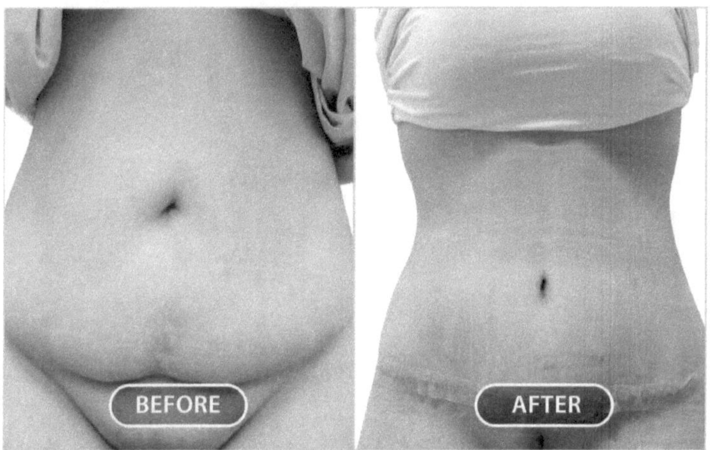

I pay attention to the umbilicus. A large umbilicus is unattractive, so it has to be made smaller. Notice the abdominal scar is positioned very low to reduce the mons pubis and lengthen the appearance of the torso.

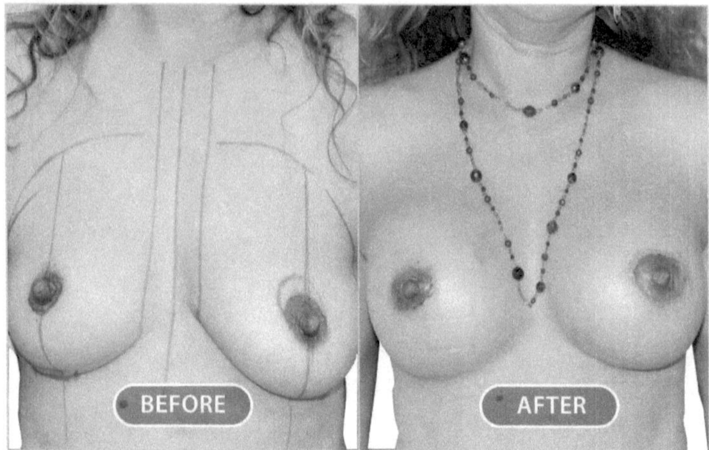

Breast augmentation through a small scar on the boarder of the areola. The left side required a mini lift to achieve better symmetry.

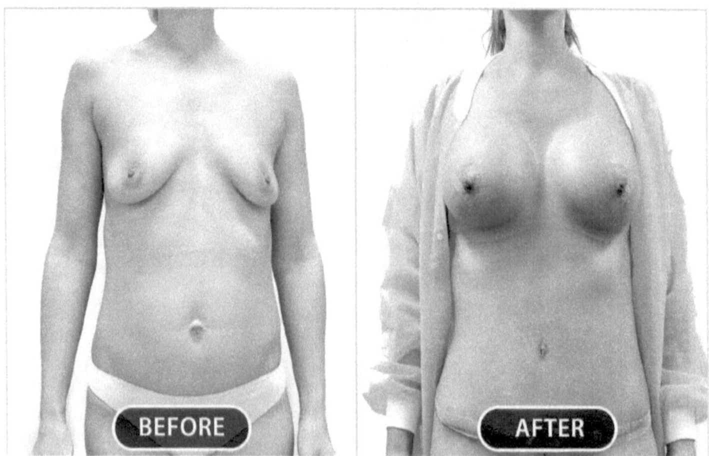

Attention to detail produces an artistic cosmetic abdominal unit, a small umbilicus, a short pubis and low scar.

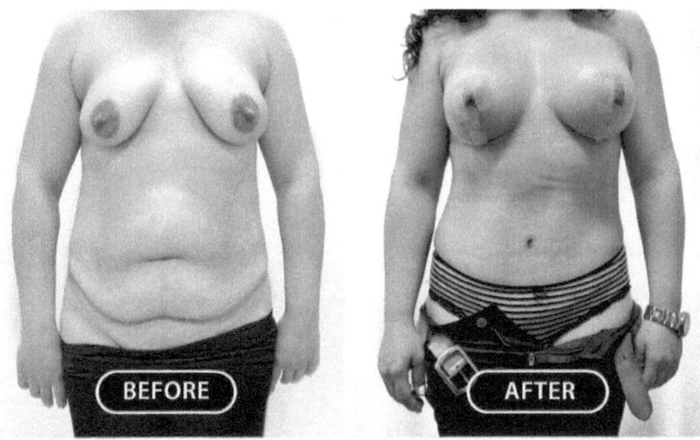

A five-hour Mummy Makeover has transformed this women's body.

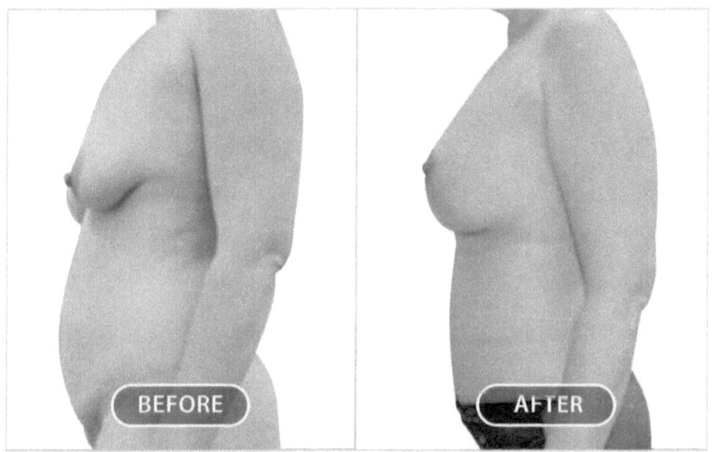

When a mummy makeover is performed properly, it is done only once in a patient's lifetime.

Arm Lift & Arm Reduction

"Lunch lady arms!" said Annie woefully as she raised her arm and jiggled her triceps area. "I'm too young to have lunch lady arms!"

After losing weight, Annie ended up with excess skin on her upper arms. "I thought when I lost weight, I would be able to wear sleeveless tops again but noooooo!" she said. The best option, given that exercise would never shrink the excess skin, was to have an arm lift and arm reduction done. This was the procedure that would give Annie the most confidence. We did it in conjunction with a few other procedures, including a tummy tuck and butt lift. Finally, Annie realised her dream of having a truly healthy-looking body, free of the excess skin of her once-heavy frame.

An arm lift and liposuction plastic surgery, or brachioplasty as it is sometimes called, is designed to remove the excess skin and fat in the upper arm, reduce the arm circumference and reshape the upper arm area.

An upper arm lift, or arm reduction, is part of a cosmetic plastic surgery procedure called "body contouring", which is designed to remove skin and fat from various body areas. This sagging skin in the upper arm is typically caused by weight loss. However, the natural ageing process also causes the skin to lose elasticity and become lax.

Arms tend to lose their firmness as the layers of muscle and supporting fat become thinner. Some call this a "batwing" deformity. In such cases, an arm lift can assist in restoring and tightening these areas, offering a much firmer, youthful look and leaving the individual more confident to wear sleeveless tops and dresses. The final scar is often unfavourable and requires scar management to improve on its quality.

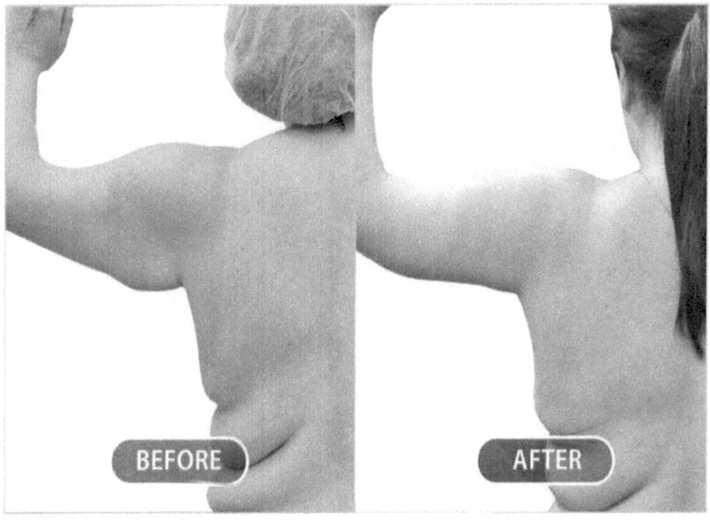

Arm reduction and liposuction.

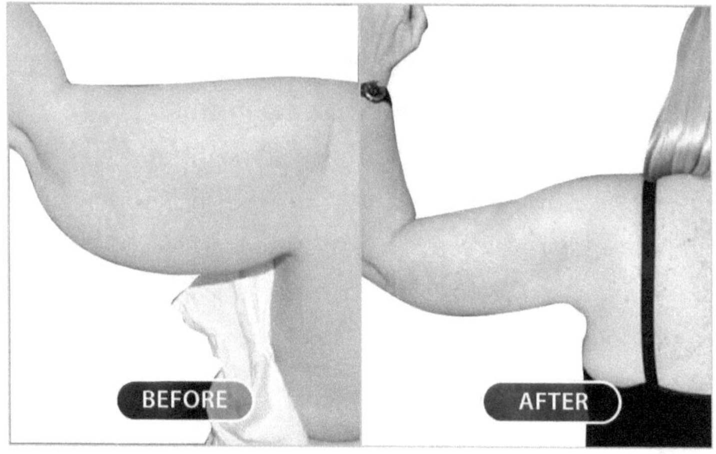

The scar is often concealed when the arms are placed by the sides.

Thigh Lift & Thigh Reduction

Sixty-one-year old Rita has been playing league tennis for most of her adult life and is extremely fit for her age. However, she had recently become self-conscious about the development of sagging in her inner thighs. "It's not a good look," she said, commenting about how her legs looked in today's short tennis skirts. She came to me for a thigh lift to tighten up the sagginess of her inner thighs. Rita was so pleased with the results that she came back for a few additional procedures, including a mini-facelift and neck lift.

Sagging skin is usually caused by weight loss, but the natural ageing process also causes the skin to lose elasticity. Both men and women often find that the thighs, in particular, lose their firmness as the layers of muscle become thinner. In such cases, a thigh lift can help to restore and tighten these areas, giving a much firmer, youthful look and leaving the patient more confident to wear fitted trousers as well as skirts and shorts.

A thigh lift is a well-tolerated procedure that can help improve the contour of the medial portion of the upper leg by removing excess skin and fatty tissue. Often combined with liposuction, this procedure can help refine the thigh to a more shapely, youthful appearance. Scarring from the thigh lift is concealed in the groin area and the inner aspect of the thigh.

During this surgery, I place the incision along the upper, inner thigh area. In some cases, where additional lift is needed, the incision may carry on along either the groin line or the buttock fold. Excess skin and fat are removed through the incision, and I stitch the remaining skin closed. Sometimes the operation is performed in conjunction with liposuction. Regardless of the location of the surgical incision, every effort is made to ensure that the resulting scars will be as inconspicuous as possible.

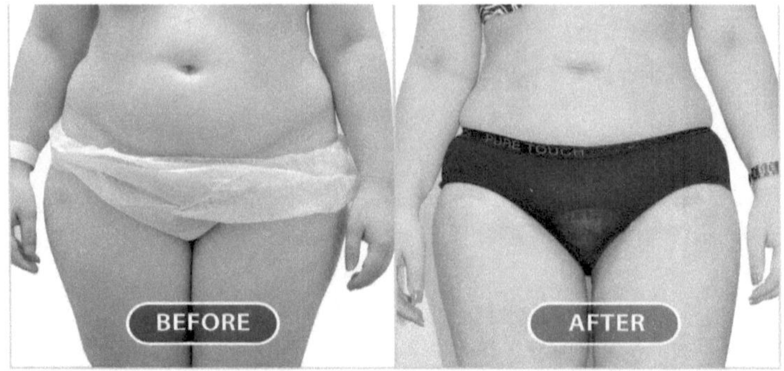

I generally prefer to do circumferential thigh liposuction and allow the skin to contract for six months. It can be followed by a thigh lift, should it be required. A two-stage procedure generally produces a shorter thigh scar than a one-stage procedure.

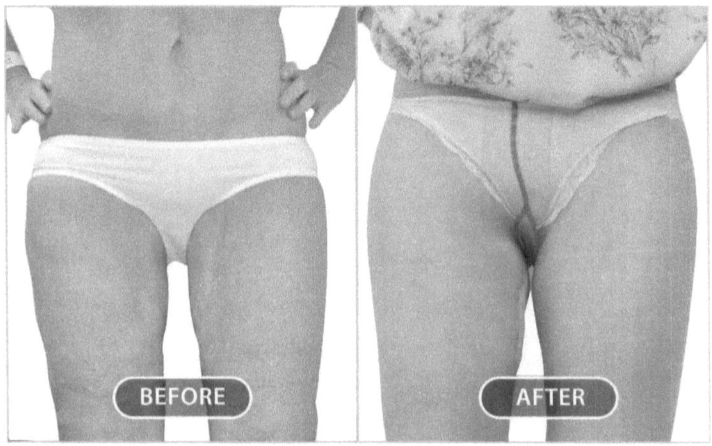

Thigh lift surgery: excessive tissue is removed and the skin tightened.

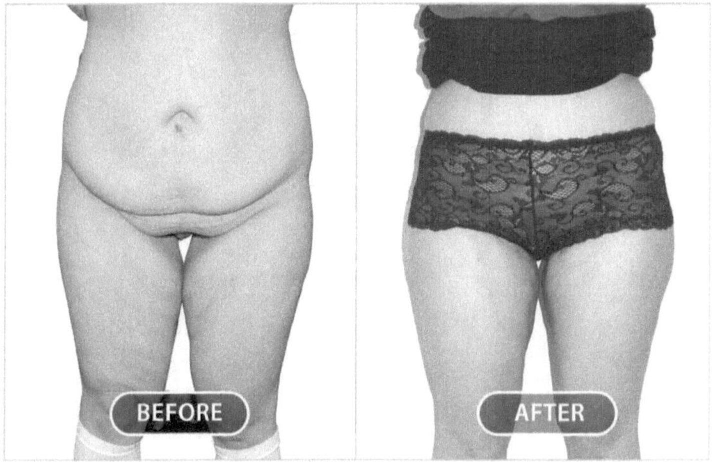

This patient had abdominoplasty and thigh lift surgery.

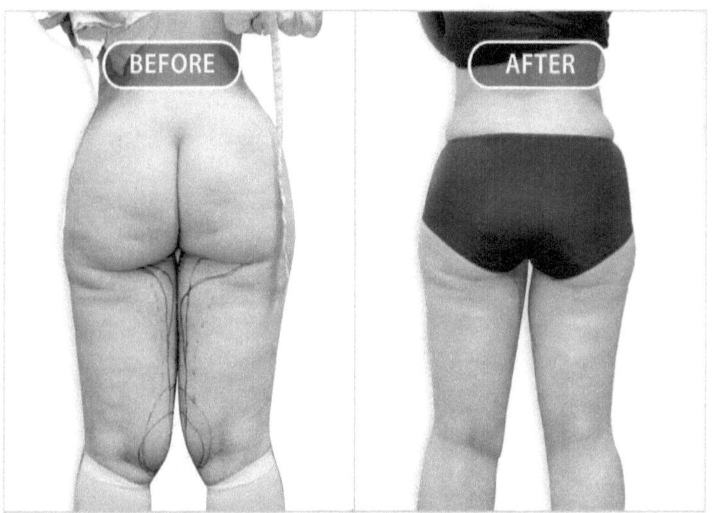

This patient had a thigh lift and liposuction.

Excessive Sweating Reduction

Mike's role as CEO meant lots of meetings with clients, board members and staff. Mike is a personable and confident fellow who is also a great leader. However, Mike had one secret that he fought daily to correct: excessive sweating in his hands, feet, and armpits. This bothered Mike because he felt that people who sweat that much are often perceived as dishonest, or that they're hiding something. He was very proud of what he had achieved as a leader and didn't want to jeopardise that with what he called "my sweat flood".

Copious applications of antiperspirants didn't solve the problem, and Mike often found himself changing his shirt and socks several times throughout the day to avoid the obvious odour and sweat stains on his clothing.

When Mike discovered that he had a treatable condition he was ecstatic. He immediately booked a treatment that involved injections of Botox into his armpits, hands and feet. The procedure was a huge success, giving Mike the confidence he needs as a leader.

Excess sweating, which is also called hyperhidrosis, is sweating beyond a level needed to maintain normal body temperature in response to heat exposure or exercise. It can have many causes including drug reactions, the use of antidepressants, underlying disease, menopause, extreme sensitivity to spicy foods or chronic stress.

Excessive sweating may be socially embarrassing and/or may interfere with certain professions. Excessive sweating in the palms (palmar hyperhidrosis) may impede artwork, working with electrical components or playing certain musical instruments. In addition, hyperhidrosis may stain clothing and necessitate several changes of clothing every day.

There are several options for treating hyperhidrosis:

- Armpit skin resection and gland debulking, also known as open adenectomy. This is a surgical procedure that is often performed under local anesthetic and sedation. It involves the removal of an ellipse of skin and sweat glands from the armpit. It creates a 4 cm scar in the hair-bearing skin in the axillae (armpit) and gives a long-lasting result.

- MiraDry® uses thermal energy to create heat in the area where bothersome sweat and odour glands reside and safely eliminates them. This is an office-based treatment, performed under local anaesthesia. It takes 45 minutes for each armpit, and most patients can return immediately to regular activity and work. You may experience swelling, numbness, bruising and sensitivity in the underarm area for several days after treatment. Exercise is typically resumed after five days. With MiraDry®, you can expect immediate and permanent results.

This treatment is cost effective and permanently reduces both odour and sweat gland secretion.

- Botox—Sweat glands need a nerve impulse to be activated. Without this stimulation, they won't secrete sweat. By injecting Botox (botulinum toxin) into problem areas such as the underarms, hands and feet, the related nerve impulse is temporarily blocked and prevented from reaching the sweat gland. This, in turn, stops sweat production in the treated area. The treatment is as simple as it sounds. All patients report a substantial reduction in sweating within two days. A repeat treatment is generally recommended within six months. An injection into the underarms and hands has been shown to be very successful. Good results can be achieved after a single treatment session and the effects last for up to six months.

CHAPTER FOUR

Buttocks Surgery

Both men and women may feel self-conscious about their buttocks and legs. In many cases, exercise and weight loss won't deliver the desired shape, but plastic surgery can offer a great deal of improvement.

Recent studies in evolutionary biology have suggested a strong correlation between the hourglass figure and overall physical and psychological health. This correlation is best summarised by an ideal waist-to-hip ratio of 0.7, so your waist width is 30 per cent narrower than your hip width. However, this ratio can vary depending on your age, race and societal trends.

It is vitally important to know that the anatomy is different for men and women. Curvy lines, round volumes and prominent projection characterise women's buttocks, while men's buttocks are characterised by straight lines, square volumes and side depressions. There should be no sagginess of the buttock nor full gluteal crease, which indicates early buttock sagginess.

Buttocks enhancement, lift and/or reshaping surgery should address these points as well as the presence of fatty fullness under the crease (what is known as the "banana roll deformity"), cellulite-contour irregularity of the skin, and saddlebags.

Different techniques suit different patients for buttock contouring surgery. These include a variety of techniques such as liposuction to sculpt the shape of the buttocks, a buttock lifting procedure and buttock augmentation procedures, using either lipofilling or implants.

The buttocks on the back play the same role as the breasts on the front. The key features of both are the projection and the curved shape that many women find desirable.

This is a relatively new field in aesthetic surgery; however, in recent times, this type of operation has become more common, particularly in big cities like Sydney, Rio de Janeiro, Miami and Los Angeles.

One of the most popular procedures is the Brazilian Butt Lift (BLL), which is another name for buttocks augmentation, or fat transfer to the buttocks. BLL employs a combination of liposculpture and fat grafting to increase the volume and enhance the shape of the buttocks.

Buttocks Augmentation

Amelia felt that her buttocks were too flat for someone as active as she was. Amelia had an athletic body, but said, "I guess I wasn't blessed with an athlete's booty". She wanted a rounder, more feminine yet powerful look that was more proportionate to the rest of her body. However, no amount of deadlifts, squats or sprints managed to build up her gluteal muscles to the shape she desired. Amelia opted for a natural look using her own fat, transplanted from her inner thighs, love handles and waist areas. The buttocks augmentation procedure gave her buttocks the rounder look she wanted and the confidence to go with an "all-around" curvy look.

Buttocks augmentation procedures alter and improve the appearance of the buttocks. Many people have small or flat buttocks that don't respond significantly to weight training. As a result, they opt to augment their buttocks with either fat transfer or implants for a more curvy look in women and a more athletic and powerful look in men. This surgery is performed in combination with liposculpture to contour the entire back area.

Also referred to as a Brazilian Butt Lift (BLL), buttocks augmentation is a procedure that employs a combination of liposculpture and fat grafting to increase the volume and enhance the shape of the buttocks. This results in enhancement of the shape, volume and gluteal area of the buttocks. It also has a lifting effect, resulting in a perkier appearance.

Individuals who desire buttocks augmentation, have two options: fat transfer, or buttock implants.

Fat transfer uses fat cells harvested from the patient's stubborn fat areas, which are then purified and transferred to the buttocks to enhance the volume, shape and/or position of their buttocks and hips. Targeted fatty cells are removed via liposuction in a sculpting fashion from stubborn problem areas, such as the inner and outer thighs, lower back, abdomen, love handles, bra rolls and/or arms. The fat cells are then prepared for grafting to the gluteal (buttocks) area to augment the contour and projection of this area. Fat transfer is generally performed under general anaesthesia. It has a quicker recovery time than augmentation with buttock implants.

More dramatic results can be achieved with implants. This procedure is a more significant operation requiring an overnight stay in hospital, but it gives permanent results. It involves a 7 cm single incision located over the tailbone in the midline, through which I introduce the implant and position it within the gluteus muscles. This is the best position for the implant as the muscle covers the implants entirely and gives a brilliant outcome.

I use implants when patients do not have sufficient fat storage and wish to achieve a "dramatic effect".

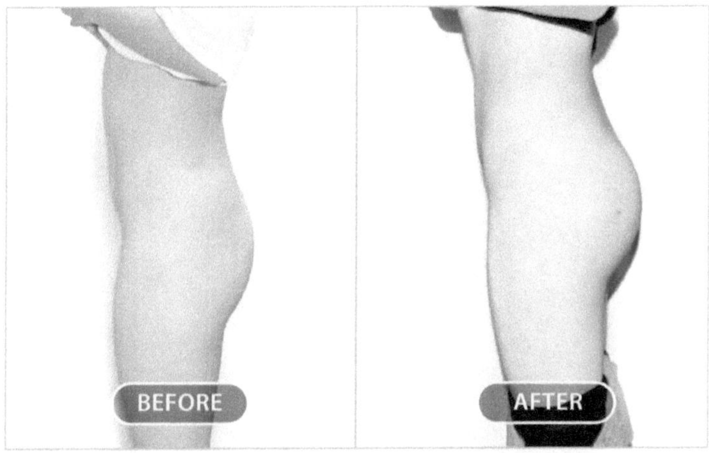

Notice the difference in this patience after she had 240cc round buttock implants.

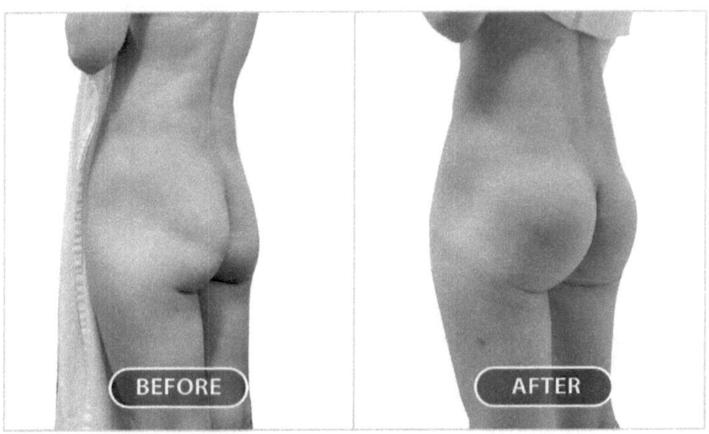

Buttock implant surgery using 280cc round implants.

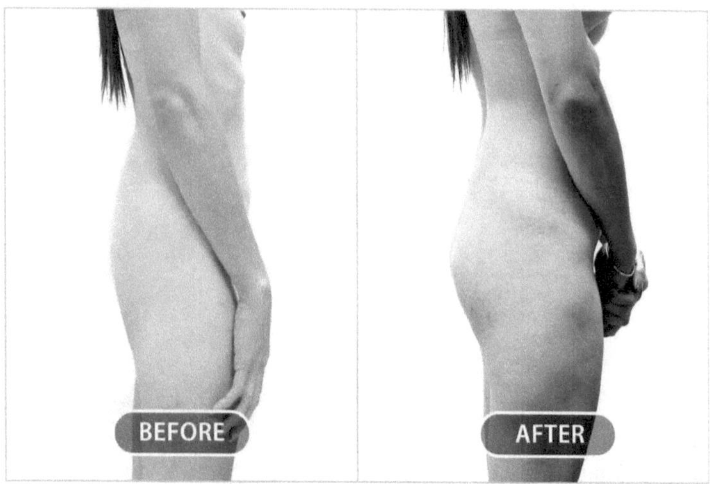

Buttock augmentation surgery, using 270cc round buttock implants.

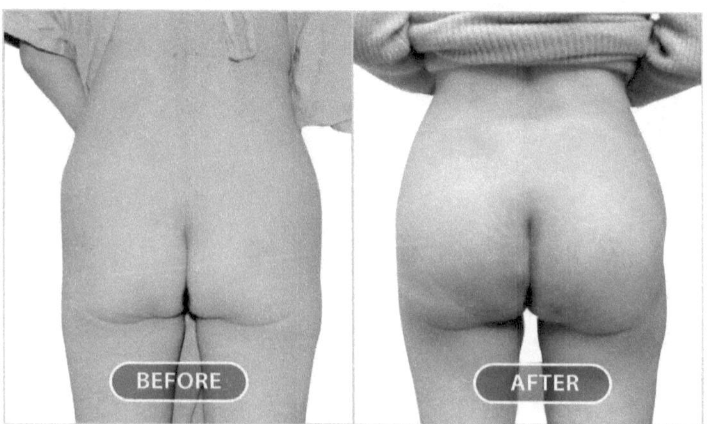

These are before and after photos of a 330cc round buttock implant procedure.

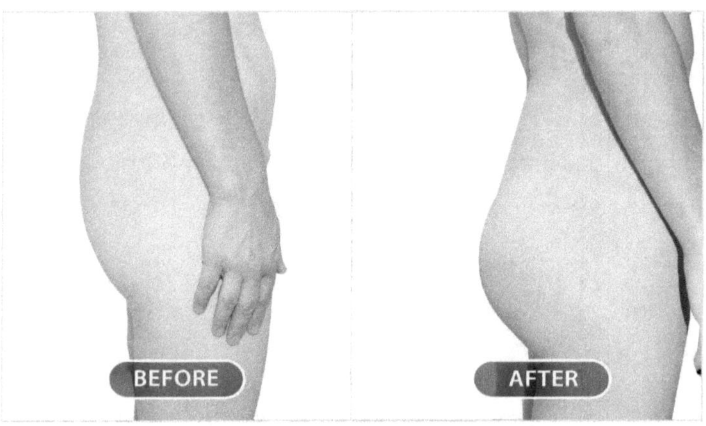

Buttock augmentation using 350 cc round implants.

Butt Lift & Reshaping

Marci had always admired women with curves, and especially curvy buttocks. Marci was not skinny, but she never had what she wanted: a curvy hourglass figure. When she attempted to gain weight to give herself a more rounded figure, the new weight never settled where she wanted it. She wanted to round out her butt but not her belly. Ultimately, Marci settled for a butt lift and reshaping, which gave her the rounded, perky butt she always dreamed of having.

Aesthetic surgery of the buttocks includes many options and combinations of methods, including: liposuction, buttock lift, buttock implants and/or fat transfer procedures. Patients with traumatic buttock injuries and contour deformities from injections also need correctional procedures, often with fat injections, and grafting of tissue flaps from another part of your body. The dramatic increase in the need for body contouring following massive weight loss (i.e. diet controlled or after bariatric surgical treatments for obesity) has extended to buttock surgery.

Flat buttock deformities caused by weight loss are often severe in nature and increase the need for a buttock lift and reshaping surgery.

Such surgery should address the whole back, flanks, hip, thighs, bra lines and waistline as one unit.

Buttock lift and reshaping surgery should also address the presence of fatty fullness under the crease (what is known as "banana roll deformity"), cellulite-contour irregularity of the skin and saddlebags.

Patients come to me with various challenges, such as:

- Small buttocks;

- Saggy buttocks;

- Flattened buttocks (developmental or post weight loss);

- Buttocks that are disproportionate to the rest of the body;

- Large buttocks and thighs;

- Large flanks; and

- Lack of waist definition.

Different techniques suit different patients, so I often use a combination of procedures to achieve the best possible outcome.

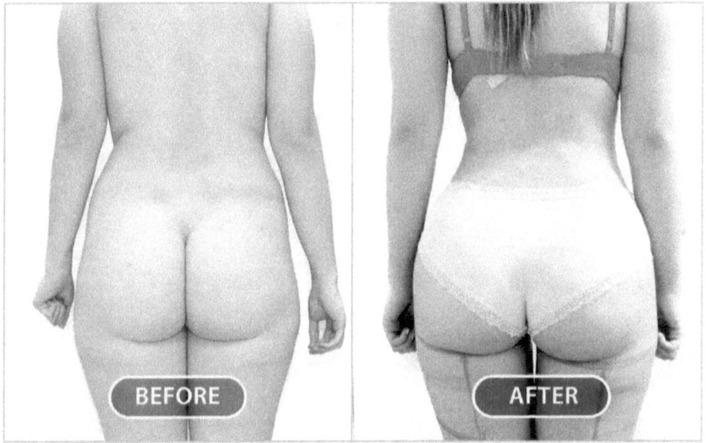

Notice the desirable gap in the inner thighs, the narrow waist, and the fully rounded buttocks that this patient has achieved after receiving her Brazilian Buttock Lift.

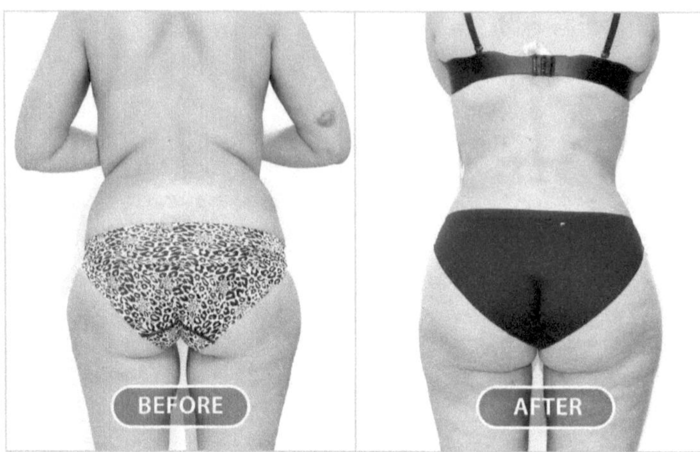

Liposuction of the inner thigh and back area define the buttocks and waistline.

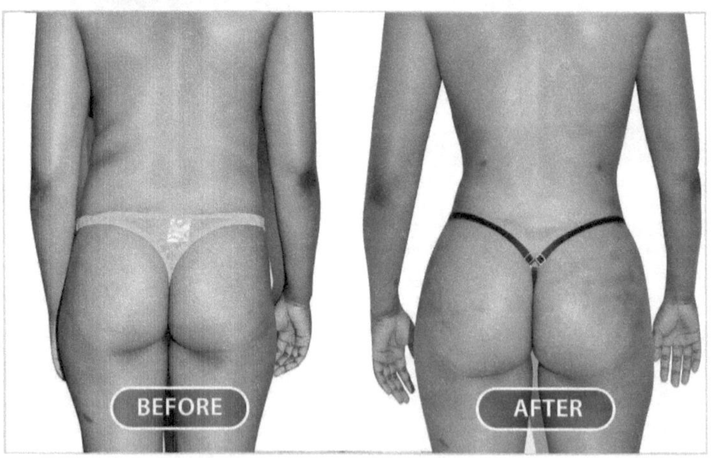

After the Brazilian Buttock Lift, which involved a fat transfer to the buttocks and liposculpture of the waistline, flanks and inner thighs.

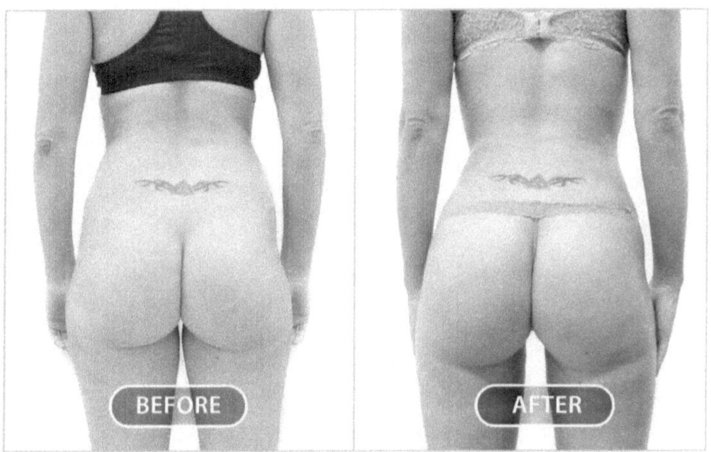

Brazillian Buttock Lift and posterior recontouring. Notice the desirable inner thighs gap, narrow waist and fat injected buttocks.

Buttocks Liposuction

"I got rid of it everywhere else, so why not my butt?" asked Laura during a consultation about her desire for buttock liposuction. She was, of course, talking about excess fat. She had recently lost weight, but despite that, she could not get rid of what she saw as a too-large butt. She wanted a more sculpted athletic look, not the wide-hipped, heavy saddlebags look that she inherited from her mother's side of the family.

"Jeans never fit me. If they fit my butt, they're massive around my legs, and if they fit my legs, I can't even pull them higher than my thighs. I just want to wear cute jeans. Is there anything I can do?" she asked me.

I introduced Laura to liposuction; and with that procedure, I helped her achieve a more balanced posterior, removing the heaviness from her buttocks and upper thighs. Today, Laura is glowing with self-esteem and confidence; and she's loving wearing her trendy skinny jeans!

Liposuction is the most commonly performed plastic surgery procedure in Australia. This technique is used to reshape the body by permanently eliminating localised fat deposits. Countless patients become disheartened at having lost unwanted weight without seeing a significant difference in this area.

The general proportions of the body may become unbalanced, and the additional volume can restrict clothes from fitting well. In these cases, liposuction can successfully trim excess fat to bring better balance and symmetry to the body. Liposuction is a great way to get rid of those bulges that are resistant to diet and exercise.

Usually, suctioning is done in the low back above the buttocks, the back of the thigh just beneath the buttock fold and on the inner and outer thigh areas.

The aim is to produce a natural rounded curve to the buttock that recalls the look of the slim, well-proportioned athletic body. The tendency to accumulate fatty deposits on the buttocks may be inherited, and these deposits are often resistant to diet and exercise.

The procedure involves making a tiny incision in the skin, usually in or near the buttock crease and then inserting a thin tube called a cannula into the fatty area. The cannula is used to break up the fat deposits and sculpt the area to the desired proportions. The unwanted fat is suctioned out with a vacuum cannula.

In the super-wet technique, a saline solution comprising a local anaesthetic and adrenaline is injected into the area to be treated, which makes the fat deposits easier to break up and extract. This extra fluid also minimises trauma to the surrounding tissue as well as reducing swelling and post-operative pain. The administration of adrenaline reduces bleeding during surgery, further reducing risks.

The tumescent technique, in which an even larger amount of liquid solution is injected, has similar benefits.

A relatively new method, called Water Jet Soft Liposuction, uses water jets to liquefy the fat and numb the area. This is followed by fat suction. Like the super-wet and tumescent techniques, the Water Jet technique minimises trauma, bruising and blood loss. It is especially useful for the removal of small and moderate amounts of fat.

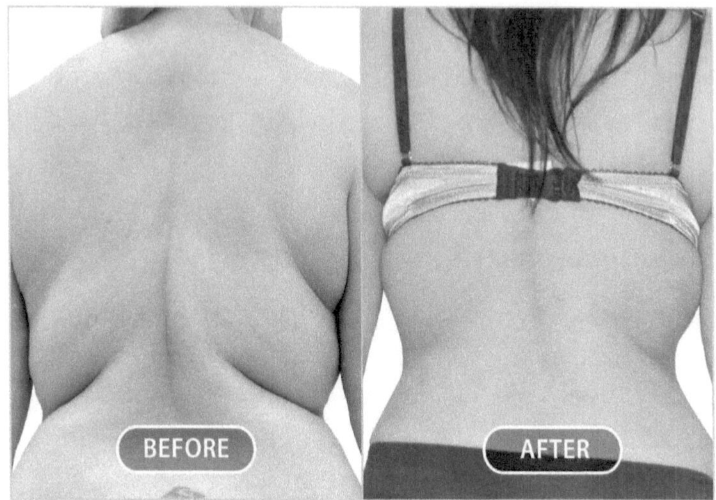

This patient had her entire back liposculptured, producing an hourglass figure.

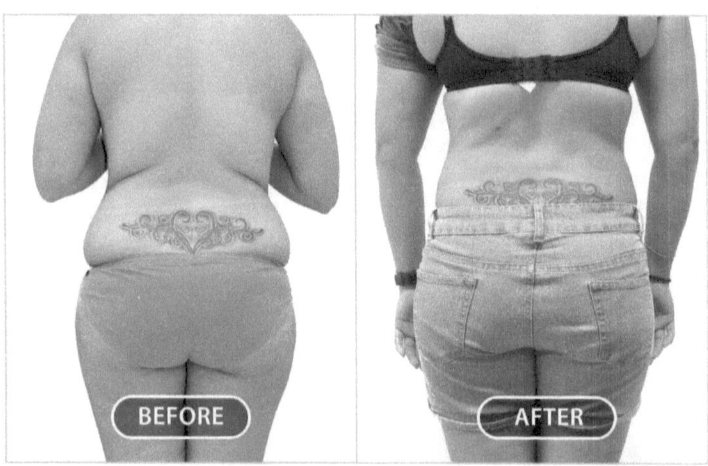

Notice how the skin folds contracted and softened by aggressive liposuction above and below the crease.

My choice of technique will be determined by a combination of factors, including: the precise area to be treated, the amount of fat to be removed and the patient's preferences.

CHAPTER FIVE

Gentital Plastic Surgery

Many men and women feel insecure about the appearance and the function of their genital areas. Problems in this part of the body can produce irritation, discomfort, avoidance of sexual activity and/or make it difficult to exercise.

A woman may have been born with saggy and lax skin in the genital area or experienced damage due to childbirth, a forceps injury, an inadequately repaired episiotomy or female mutilation.

The effects of ageing, weight loss, weight gain and/ or menopause may have taken their toll on a woman and resulted in an unwanted appearance and lack of function of the genital areas.

Those conditions can now be treated in the specialist field of female genital plastic surgery, which is also known as "aesthetic genital surgery" and includes:

- Labia minora reduction (inner labiaplasty);

- Labia majora remodelling (outer labiaplasty);

- Labial fat injection;

- Clitoral hood reduction;

- Vaginoplasty (also known as pelvic floor muscle repair and reconstruction);

- Laser vaginal rejuvenation (LVR);

- Pubic liposuction;

- Pubic lift;

- Monsplasty (mons pubis liposuction with or without a pubic lift); and

- Female genital mutilation repair surgery.

The appearance and function of female genitalia can be restored through a variety of procedures, collectively known as "vaginal rejuvenation procedures".

There are also male genital plastic surgery procedures available and these are discussed in **Chapter 6: Plastic Surgery for Men**.

Labiaplasty

Labiaplasty is a surgical procedure that is designed to alter irregularities in the appearance of, and reduce the size of, the labia. Surgery to the inner vaginal lips (inner labiaplasty) is much more common than surgery to the outer vaginal lips (outer labiaplasty).

The most common irregularity corrected by labiaplasty is reducing the size and improving the shape of inner labia that are too big. If the inner labia protrude far beyond the outer labia, there is a risk of chafing, and some women also find it is aesthetically displeasing.

I routinely perform labiaplasty surgery as day surgery under general anaesthetic. I remove a wedge-shaped piece of tissue from the labia and re-attach the labium in a new position so that the inner lips no longer protrude beyond the outer lips. If required, I also reduce the size of the clitoral hood.

I use re-absorbable stitches during labiaplasty, so the stitches do not need to be removed from this sensitive area. Recovery from labiaplasty is usually quick and easy. Sexual relations can be resumed four weeks after the procedure.

1. Female genital plastic surgery procedures – which includes labiaplasty, vaginoplasty and vaginal rejuvenation – are evidence-based medicine and research-proven treatments.

2. However, the media and public have positioned vaginal plastic surgery as procedures only undergone for aesthetic purposes, based on unrealistic female images. In fact, there was discussion in the United Kingdom at one stage to have the procedure labelled as "genetical mutilation".

3. Despite the stigma surrounding female genital plastic surgery procedures, they have become increasingly common in recent years, driven by various factors such as cultural influences, aesthetic preferences and concerns about the appearance and functionality of the female sexual organs.

4. From a global perspective, there were 194,086 labiaplasty procedures performed in 2022, which represents a 32 per cent increase over the 132,664 labiaplasties performed in 2018. The dramatic increase in the number of vaginal procedures performed over a similar period has made it one of the fastest growing areas of aesthetic plastic surgery. Figures from International Surveys of Aesthetic/Cosmetic Procedures conducted by the International Society of Aesthetic Plastic Surgeons (ISAPS).

5. There were 264,741 female genital plastic surgery procedures performed worldwide in 2022, according to the International Society of Aesthetic Plastic Surgery (ISAPS). This included 194,086 labiaplasty procedures and 70,645 vaginal rejuvenation procedures.

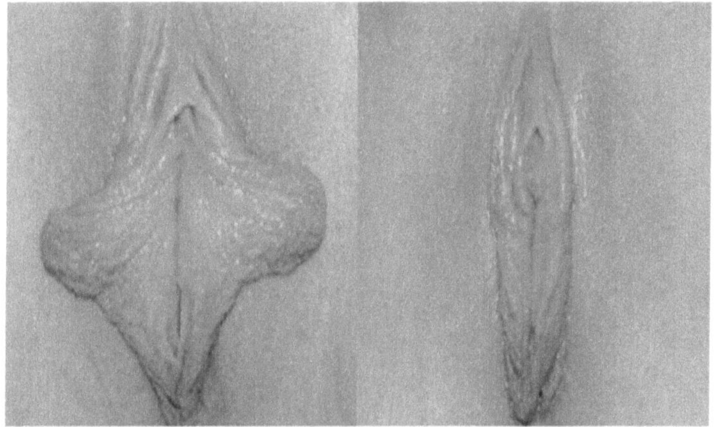

Before and after inner labiaplasty.

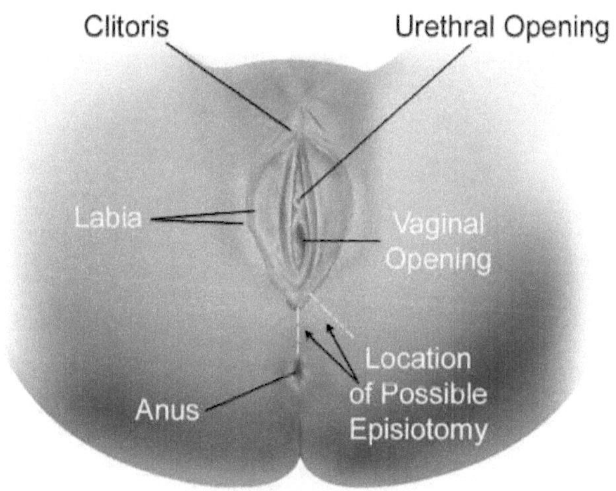

Female Perineum

Understanding the anatomy of the genital area is vital for successful surgery.

Vaginoplasty

Vaginoplasty, also known as pelvic floor reconstruction, is vaginal surgery to tighten the muscles of the pelvic floor and the vagina. It is a restorative procedure.

Childbirth can cause the vagina and pelvic floor muscles to become enlarged or stretched. Some women suffer from a stretched vagina and pelvic floor muscles after a single birth, and others after giving birth to several children. This problem can lead to a lack of structural support and uterine prolapse. Some women also feel it negatively affects their sex lives. Others report worsening of urinary stress incontinence, i.e. urine leakage due to physical movement, coughing or sneezing putting pressure on the bladder.

Post-menopausal women and women who have been treated for cervical cancer may also find their vaginas have enlarged and may request vaginoplasty.

During the vaginoplasty procedure, problems are corrected by reconstructing the vaginal and pelvic floor muscles to create a tighter vagina and prevent sagginess of the uterus. It will also prevent prolapse of the uterus, so there is anecdotal evidence that this procedure minimises the risk of urinary incontinence.

The main objective of vaginoplasty is to give women greater gratification and satisfaction during sex because they feel more friction.

Vaginoplasty takes one-and-a-half to two hours to perform. It is usually completed as day surgery, or it may require an overnight stay.

During the vaginoplasty procedure, I remove a section of the vaginal lining and reposition the underlying muscles in such a way that the outer and inner parts of the vagina are noticeably tighter.

I remove a large ellipse of tissue from the wall of the vagina, which is the weakest part of the vagina. This is the elastic tissue that is stretched and sometimes has been cut or torn during childbirth. I then reconstruct and repair the perineal and pelvic floor muscles, and finally, I reconstruct the mucosa, or vaginal lining, with re-absorbable sutures.

As well as labiaplasty and vaginoplasty, various other procedures can be performed to improve the appearance, tone, and sensation of the vagina, such as labia majora reduction (also known as outer labiaplasty), labia majora fat injection, pubic liposuction and pubic lift.

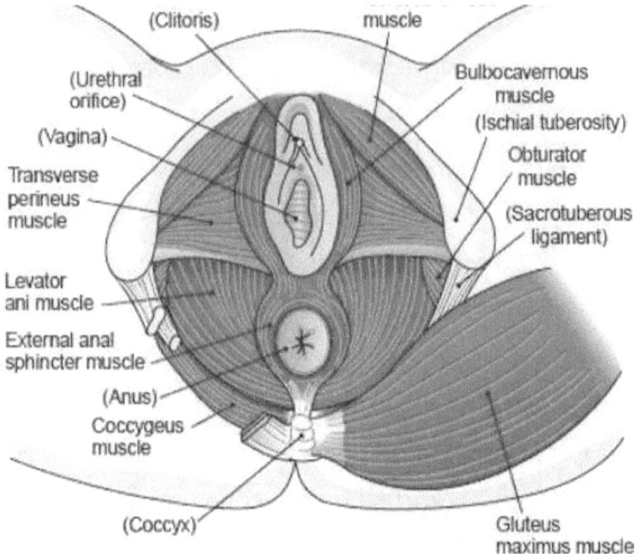

Vaginal relaxation syndrome (VRS) is a condition that medically involves the vagina and its loss of structure in women after child birth as well as due to the ageing process. Treatment for the condition includes use of surgery (surgical vaginaplasty, which is also known as pelvic floor muscle restoration surgery).

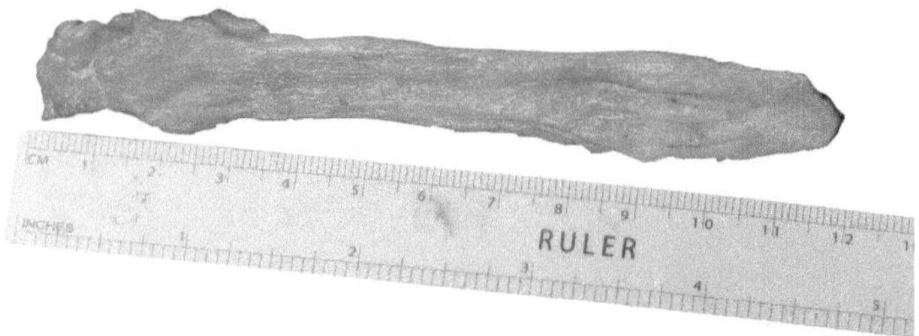

The entire amount of tissue I routinely remove from the posterior vaginal wall and perineum is around 3.5 cm x 12 cm. I would then restore the pelvic floor muscle. The entire vaginal tract and introitus is restored to its pre-labor state. I tend to over tighten the tract by 5-to-10 per cent, as the scar tends to relax and stretch six weeks post-surgery (just like any other scar in the body). Note: the average length of the vagina is 9.6 cm. I tend to remove around 3.5 x 2 cm from the perineal area and 3.5 x 10 cm from the entire tract.

Vaginal Rejuvenation Laser

The versatile nature of laser has been implemented as a modality for vaginal rejuvenation that heralds a new era of fractional CO_2 vaginal rejuvenation. This procedure produces a tighter, more elastic and rejuvenated vagina. It also treats vaginal dehydration and painful sexual intercourse (dyspareunia), remodels the vaginal mucosa, reduces vaginal atrophy and improves stress urinary incontinence.

The laser lightens the colour of the labia to enhance its appearance and give it a natural and silky texture. It also reduces wrinkles and tightens labial skin, making it more elastic.

The 20-minute procedure is minimally invasive and involves no anaesthesia, no incision, no bleeding and no shaving.

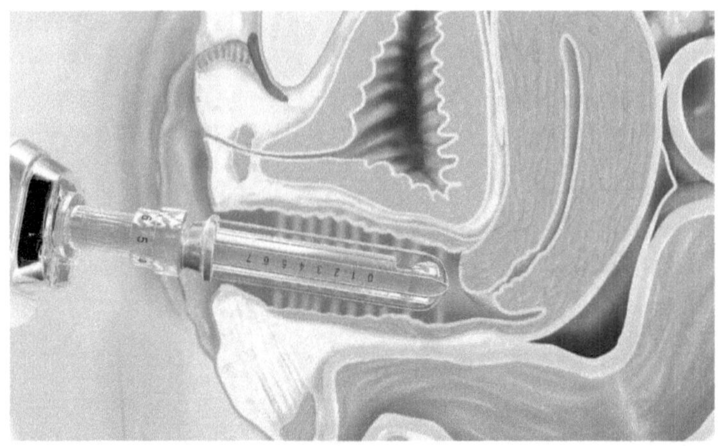

Insertion of the vaginal laser.

> → Vaginal laser is ideal due to the fact that it helps to bring back the ideal vaginal PH and deals with symptoms such as atrophy, dryness, and irritation, among other problematic issues found with ageing.
>
> → Laser Vaginaplasty restores the structure of your mucosa. The procedure takes 20 minutes to perform, requires no anaesthesia, and is not painful. You can drive in and out.
>
> → There is no down time, and you will be back to form within five days and be able to resume normal sexual activity.

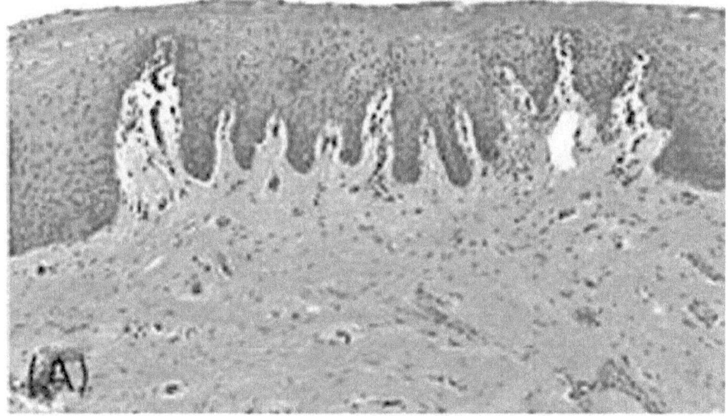

Before vaginal laser, notice the vaginal mucosa tissue atrophy, characterised by thinner epithelium and presence of papillae.

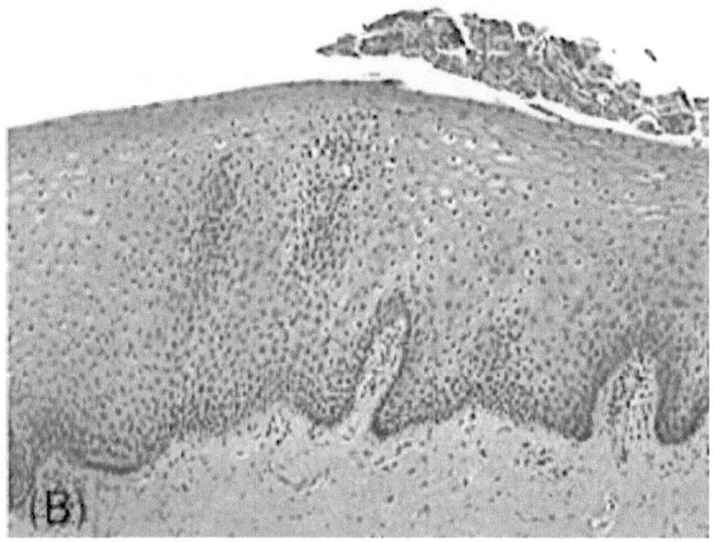

One month after vaginal laser, notice how much thicker the epithelium is. Notice also the shedding of big cells from the free surface together with a larger diameter of the epithelial cells rich in glycogen, demonstrating a restored epithelium.

Mons Pubis Surgery

Bridget is a bodybuilder, who has no noticeable fat on her body, with the exception of her mons pubis. She underwent pubic liposuction. The procedure has significantly improved this area of her body and given her greater self-confidence on the stage.

Some women struggle with a bulge of excess skin and fat in the mons, the upper part of the hair-bearing part of their vulva. Women can accumulate more fat than usual in their pubic mound with age, after childbirth or due to obesity. The bulge can result in women feeling too embarrassed to wear a bathing suit or tight pants.

The purpose of a mons pubis surgery, which is also called monsplasty, is to reduce the amount of fatty tissue and/or skin, depending on the cause of the bulge. This procedure involves mons pubis liposuction with or without a pubic lift and results in a lower profile mons that typically projects less in clothing. In some patients with a mons that hangs, removal of excess skin and a pubic lift results in less hanging. A good mons pubis lift and/ or liposuction can last a lifetime if you maintain a healthy and consistent weight following surgery.

Mons Pubis Liposuction

Mons pubis liposuction can be performed alone depending on the concerns and anatomy of the patient. Sometimes it is combined with a pubic lift and abdominoplasty (tummy tuck) procedure. Modern liposuction techniques are minimally invasive, requiring only a small incision to insert the cannula and remove unwanted fat from the area.

Mons Pubis Lift

This is a surgical procedure which requires a general anaesthetic and therefore carries a longer recovery time than liposuction alone. The procedure will be tailored to the specific shape and concerns of the patient. The operation usually takes about 60–90 minutes. I normally perform it in conjunction with mons pubis liposuction to optimise the outcome.

Some women combine a mons pubis lift with labiaplasty, a full vaginal rejuvenation or as part of a mummy makeover surgery.

With liposuction alone, the patient requires only three days off work. If you are doing both liposuction and a pubic lift, then plan for five-to-seven days recovery time.

It may take from two-to-three weeks for swelling and bruising to subside. Excess tumescent fluid may seep through the tiny incision for a few days after the procedure, and a compression garment is usually worn.

Patients may also feel tender and tight in the area for a few days after the surgery. You are encouraged to go back to light duties and work within 48 hours of having the liposuction procedure on the mons pubis.

While complications are rare, they can include bleeding, haematoma, infection and scarring.

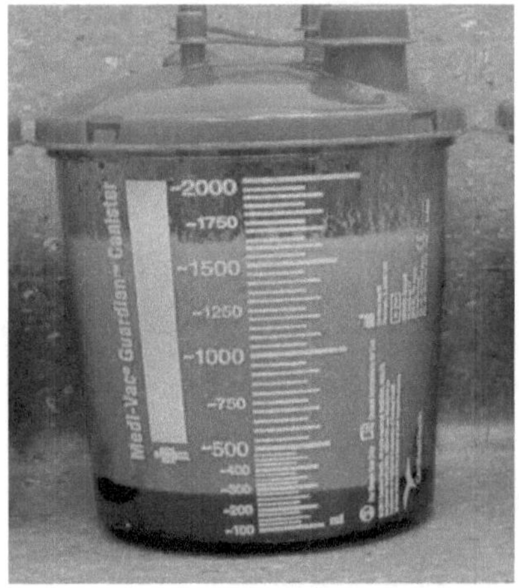

Up to 1.5L can be liposuctioned from the mons pubis and lower abdomen.

CHAPTER SIX

Plastic Surgery for Men

Men too, look in the mirror and make a list of their imperfections. These include: crow's feet and frown lines, saggy neck skin, puffy eyelids, big noses, ears that stick out too far from the side of the heads, beer bellies, muffin tops and love handles, among many other things.

While some men like to age gracefully, others refuse to accept the physiological changes and prefer to do something about them.

Ten years ago, men accounted for around 15 per cent of my patients requesting cosmetic surgery procedures. This percentage has more than doubled over the last four years. Plastic surgery for men has never been more safe, available and affordable.

Scalp Reduction

Male scalp reduction surgery involves the surgical removal of parts of the already bald scalp. This is followed by the stretching of the parts of the scalp that still have new hair growth. Following stretching, the scalp is then moved to a higher position on the head.

This procedure may be recommended before hair grafting in order to leave a smaller bald area, which needs fewer hair grafts to cover it.

Suitable candidates for this procedure are patients with excellent hair on the sides and back of the scalp that can be stretched upward to cover the bald scalp, which is incised and removed.

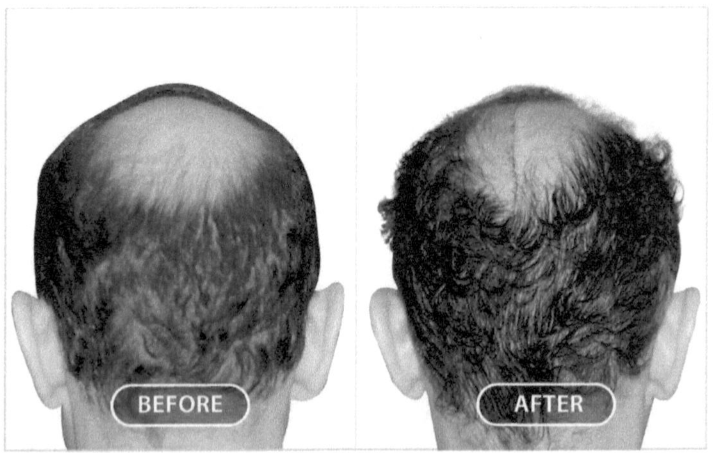

Before and after scalp reduction surgery.

Scalp reduction is usually performed using general anaesthesia, or local anaesthetic along with a sedative to aid in relaxation and reduce anxiety. Usually, a wide portion of the scalp can be removed in one session. Some patients require two-to-three sessions to achieve the coverage of hair they want.

I employ several manoeuvres, such as scoring of a tough connective tissue layer of the scalp, called the galea and wide undermining so that I can advance more tissue and remove a wider bald area. When performed properly, this technique produces a face and brow lifting effect that patients tend to enjoy as an additional benefit of scalp reduction.

Abdominal Etching

"I was tired of the 'dad bod' I had developed since my two children were born," says Ethan. "What's really nagging at me is that overall I'm still pretty fit looking. I have good legs, great arms, I'm in good shape, but I can't lose that gut, and it makes me feel like a beached whale."

Ethan, who is 45 years old, came to me with one desire: to get rid of the gut and give him a six-pack abdomen. An avid cyclist and basketball player, Ethan was certainly in good shape. Like many men in their forties, though, he had developed a belly that was resistant to exercise.

After I performed high definition (Hi Def) liposculpture and abdominal etching to give the appearance of six-pack abs, Ethan said he looked like he did in his twenties, before he became a dad, i.e. lean and fit. He started dressing in more trendy and well-fitting clothes. His new confidence and positive attitude caught the eye of his boss, who promoted him to regional sales manager.

Ethan now enjoys a more youthful look – and it has not gone unnoticed by his wife!

Known as high definition (Hi Def) abdominal liposculpture, this procedure is intended to remove excess fat from the stomach area, produce a desirable six-pack appearance and create stronger muscle definition.

I make small incisions in the belly button and the natural creases of the abdomen. I then use a hollow tube-like instrument called a cannula to, first, inject local anesthetic fluid and, then, to extract surplus fat. The fat is removed in only particular areas.

In abdominal etching, the plastic surgeon sculpts grooves in the abdominal fat layers to emphasis the abdomen's muscular contours. It's a delicate process that requires the use of liposuction to remove pockets of unwanted fat from different areas of the body.

Generally, the surgery takes about two hours and is performed under general anaesthesia as day surgery.

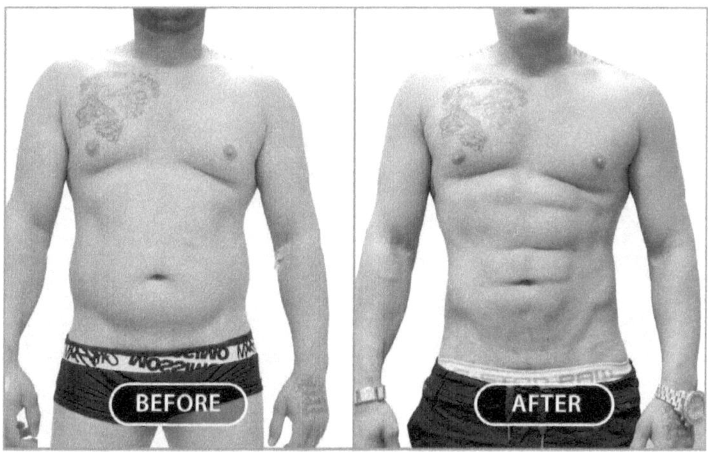

Before and after a six-pack abs surgery and chest liposculpture.

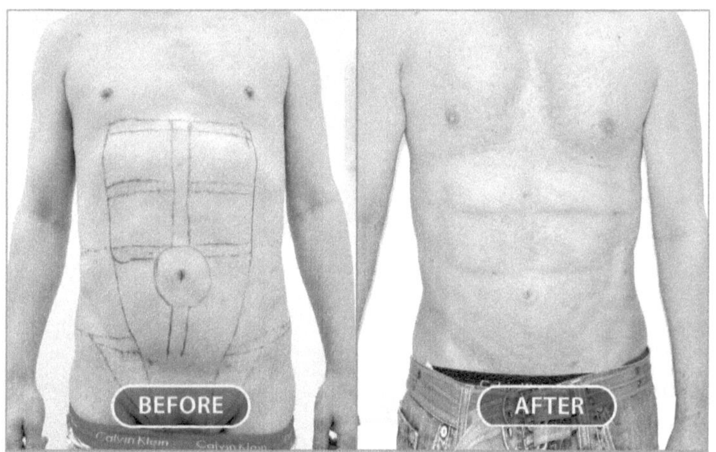

This patient had abdominal etching and pectoral implants.

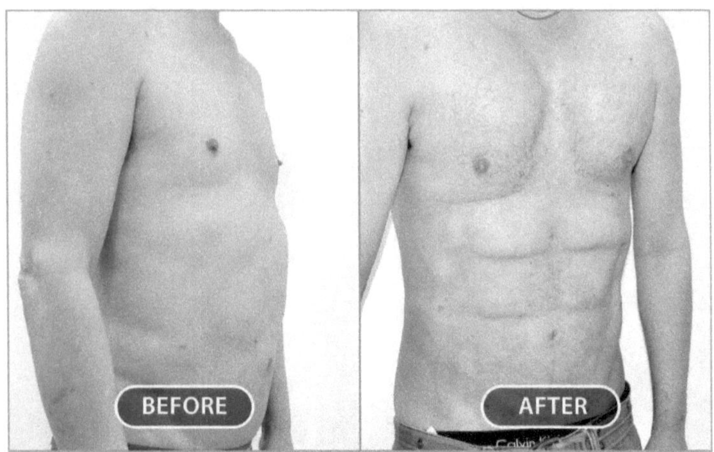

Notice the well defined six-pack created by liposculpture.

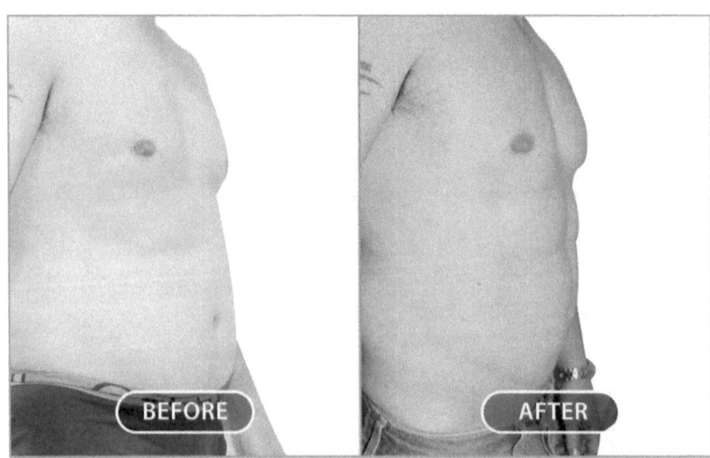

The after picture is the patient seven years after having an abdominal etching. This patient has maintained nice results.

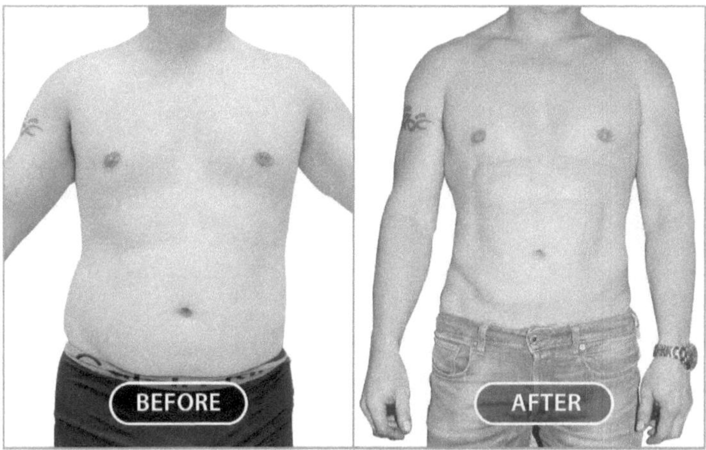

Notice the narrower waist and small belly button.

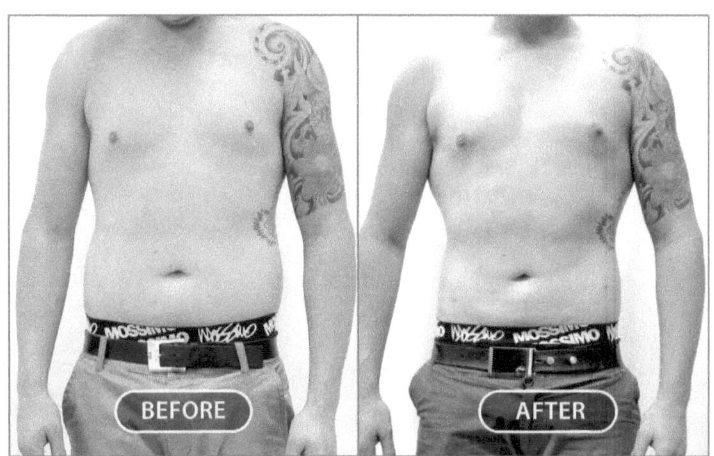

Some patients prefer a V shape. This can be achieved by liposculpturing the abdomen, hips, love handles and chest to create a V-shaped figure.

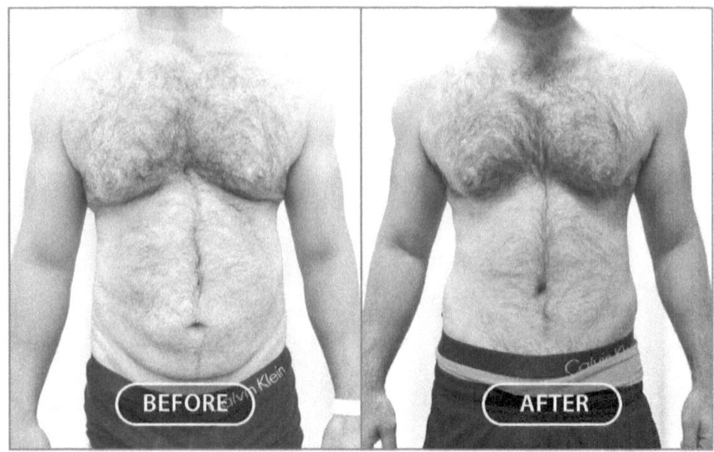

This patient underwent a full abdominoplasty and chest contouring liposculpture.

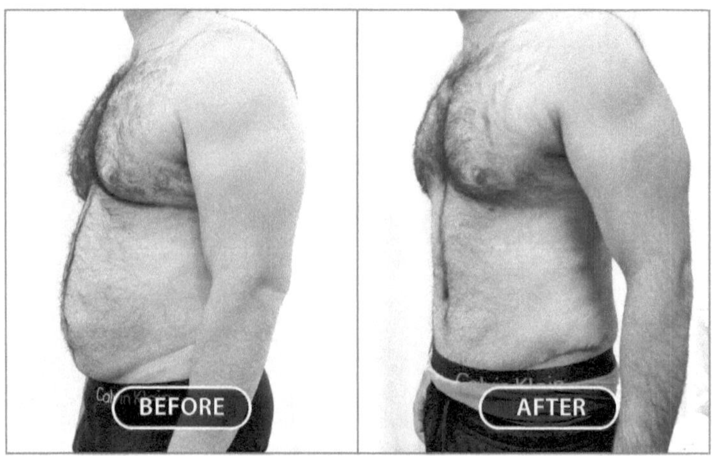

This is a natural masculine outcome.

Pectoral Enhancement

Lewis had always been very slender, and no amount of weight training ever gave him the chiselled look he was after. He had more of a marathon runner's build with a scrawny chest that never seemed to bulk up and give him the "manly" chest muscles he wanted.

Lewis was working as a lifeguard, which meant lots of time spent exposing his chest. Because he was unhappy about his looks, he often wore a baggy rashguard. This prompted teasing from his fellow lifeguards who dubbed him "stick insect".

When Lewis found out that pectoral implants were an option, he resisted. He ramped up his weight training regimen, but after six months of significantly higher intensity resistance training, his chest remained as slender as ever.

Finally, he scheduled a consultation. I explained his options and showed him before and after pictures. Somewhat reluctantly, because he was terrified of surgery, Lewis agreed to pectoral implants. Since he had little body fat to transfer and wasn't keen on a dramatic change that would leave people asking a lot of questions, we opted for relatively subtle silicone implants that would give his pectorals the definition he wanted, without appearing disproportionate to the rest of his body.

Lewis was thrilled with the results. He's still as slender as ever, but an increased dedication to his weight training has given his body an overall tone he's pleased with. Knowing that he has the "pecs to back it up", as he says, has given him unprecedented confidence.

Many men are unhappy with the natural size of their chests. They may have poorly defined pectoral muscles or wish to correct an imbalance in pectoral size or shape. If exercise (specifically, weightlifting) doesn't correct the issue, plastic surgery can help.

Pectoral enhancement is a surgical procedure used to improve the size and shape of a man's chest and provide pectoral muscle definition.

I generally perform this surgery with general anaesthesia and there are two options to consider:

- Using the patient's own fatty tissue – I typically perform this procedure through a keyhole incision. It's less invasive than a silicone implant procedure. The procedure takes one to one-and-a-half hours and will leave a tiny 5 mm scar on the side of the chest area.

- Implant procedure – I make a 4 cm incision in the armpit or, more rarely, in the crease where the pectoral muscle meets the chest. The location will depend on the patient's anatomy and the type of implant selected.

Working through this incision, I lift the pectoral tissue and skin to create a pocket, normally right behind the pectoral muscle. I then center the implants in the ideal position where they're not readily visible or detectable by casual palpation (massage).

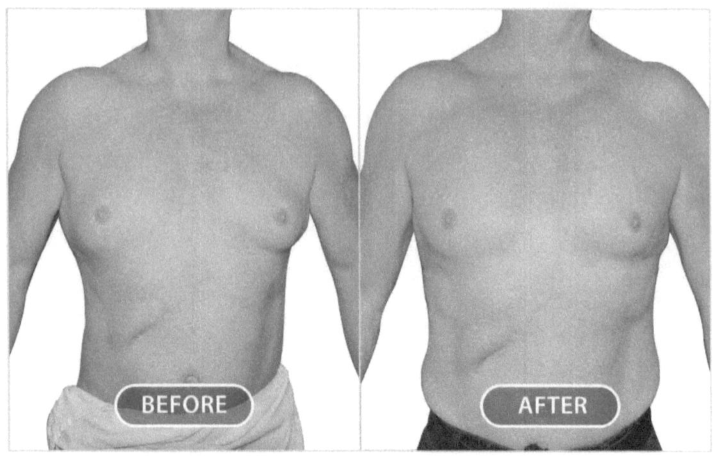

This patient had a pectoral enhancement with implants.

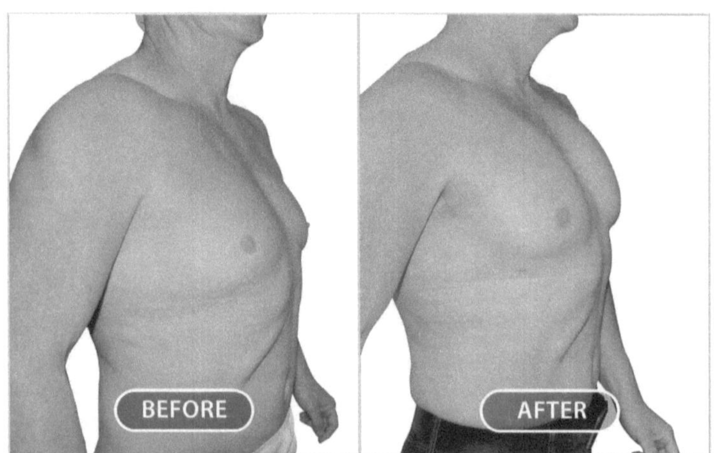

Notice the six-week old scar in the armpit.

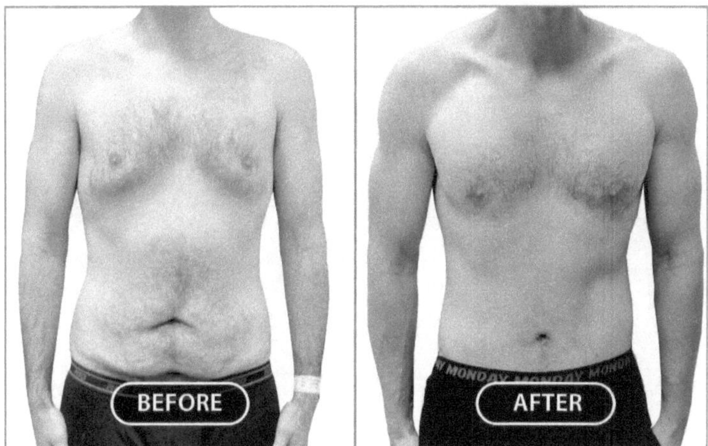

This is a patient after receiving a tummy tuck and pectoral implants.

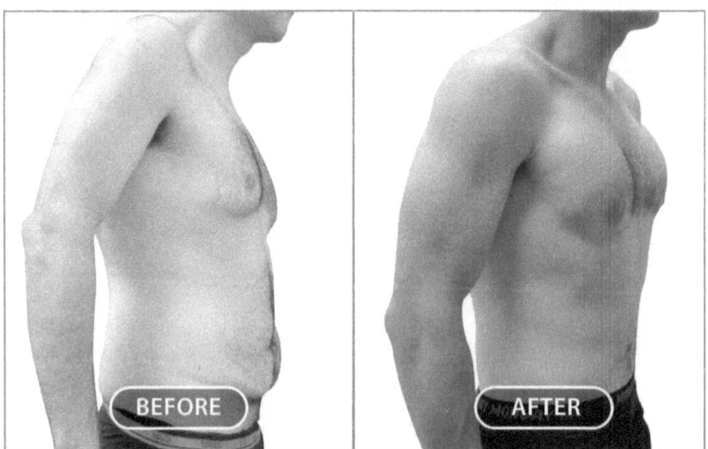

Notice the fullness of the implants at the upper pole. The size of the pectoral implants are proportionate to the rest of his body.

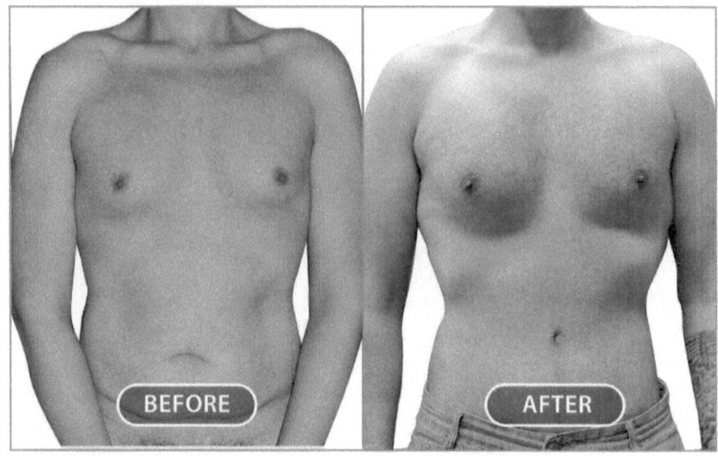

Tummy tuck and pectoral implants.

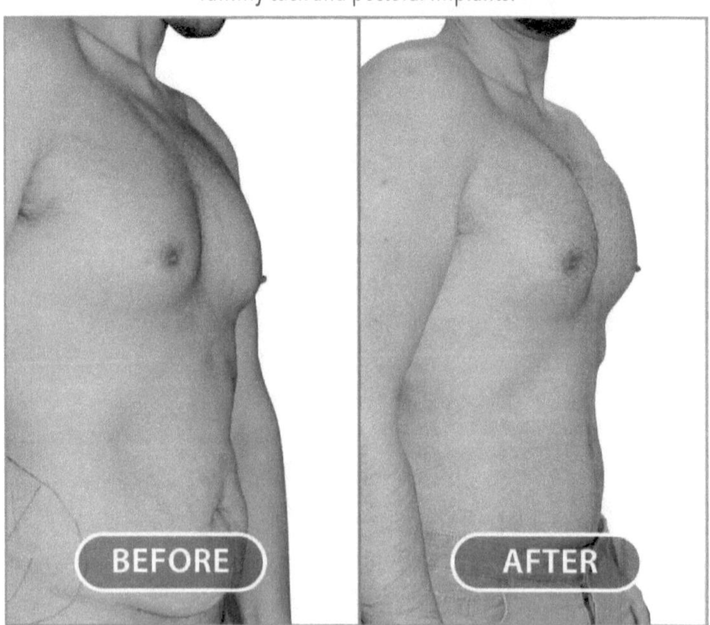

High profile pectoral implants.

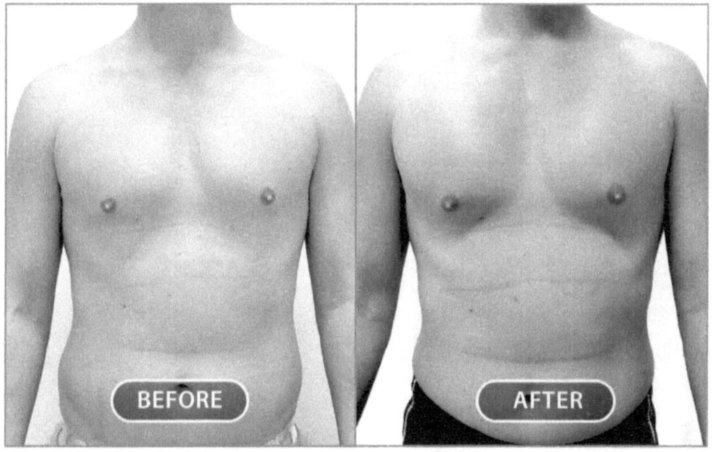

Natural-looking pectoral implants.

Male Breast Reduction

"Whatever I did, I couldn't lose the boobs," complained Greg. "Yoga, weights, running, Tai Chi… still boobs."

Greg had tried several approaches, including testosterone injections, with little success.

"There were other complications with the injections, so I stopped… and still, boobs."

Greg felt extremely uncomfortable removing his shirt in public. Even during sex, Greg preferred to keep a t-shirt on. A male friend recommended he consider breast reduction surgery. Greg's reply: "I didn't know guys could do that!" Nevertheless, he booked a consultation, and I performed a breast reduction.

Today, Greg is confident in having a masculine chest that doesn't need to be covered up.

Due to genetics or hormonal imbalances, some men develop excess tissue in their breasts. This is a condition called gynaecomastia, which is more commonly known as "man boobs".

With gynaecomastia, there is more male breast tissue than desired, resulting in a more feminine chest. This condition, which can be caused by several different things, can usually be treated successfully through male breast reduction surgery.

The 90-minute surgical procedure involves making a small incision around the lower half of the areola (nipple). I then remove the breast tissue under the nipple through this incision. The next stage is full chest liposuction to reduce and recontour the chest. Finally, I suture the incisions with dissolving sutures.

The stitches are normally located around the lower half of the areola to make the scar blend in nicely at the margins of the areola and become virtually undetectable over time.

Small "man boobs" can sometimes be reduced through a little stab incision via a liposuction procedure, such as Vaser® Liposuction or MicroAire® Liposuction.

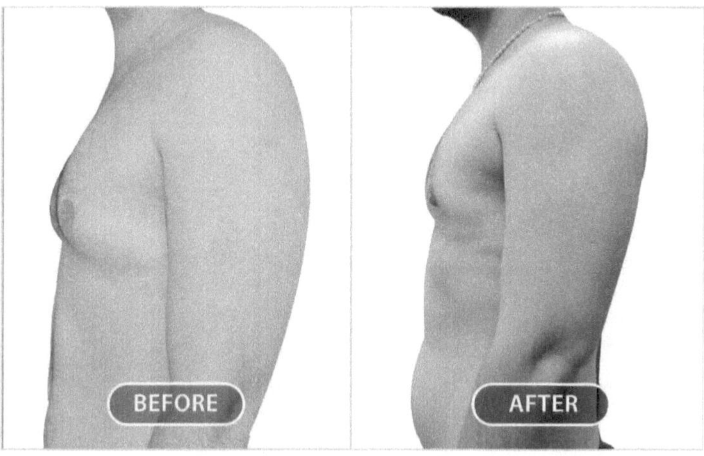

Liposuction is used to remove the fatty tissue and gynecomastia surgery to reduce the breast tissue.

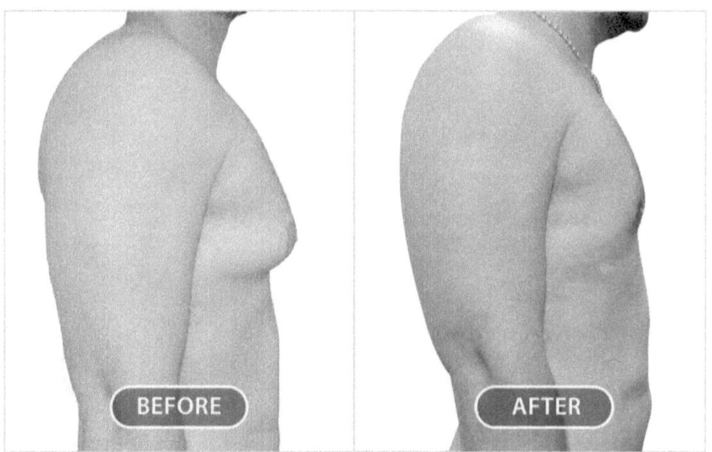

Before and after the removal of breast and fatty tissue.

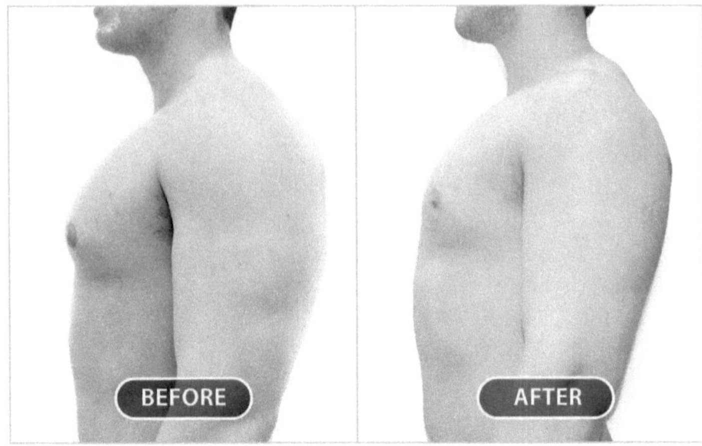

This patient had male breast reduction surgery.

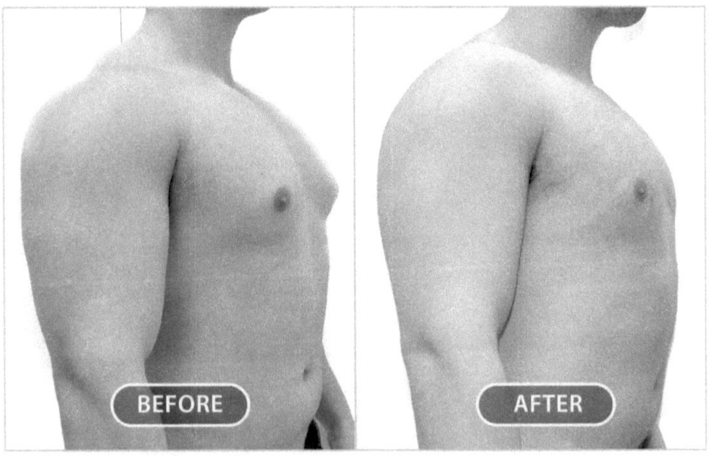

Removal of breast and fatty tissue mainly from the lower half of the chest.

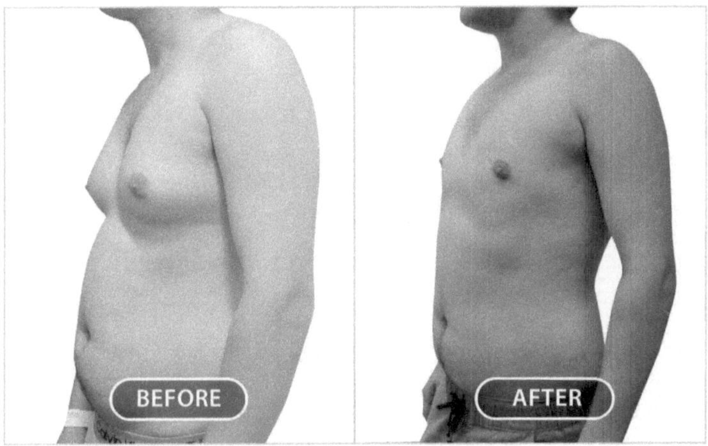

Male breast reduction and chest liposuction.

Biceps & Triceps Enhancement

After injuring his left arm in an automobile accident, Stephen suffered from nerve and tendon injury. After extensive physical therapy, he was able to regain most of the function in his arm. However, he found it impossible to restore the shape of his bicep and tricep muscles. As a result, Stephen opted to have implants inserted so that he could achieve symmetry in his arms. He is continuing with his rehabilitation. In the meantime, the surgery has given him confidence that the accident hasn't left him permanently disfigured.

Biceps and triceps enhancement is a cosmetic plastic surgery procedure that enhances the muscular appearance and improves fullness in the upper arm. This procedure is useful for patients who have nerve injury, muscle injury, tendon injury or were born with congenital abnormalities. It's also useful in both amateur or professional bodybuilders who find it difficult to tone their bicep or tricep muscles.

The enhancement can be achieved by either using fat injections or by using silicone implants. Two types of silicone implants are available for biceps and triceps implants: soft silicone and hard silicone implants.

In the case of fat transplants, it is most common for the fat cells to be taken from the buttocks, stomach or thighs of the patient. This is usually performed by liposuction. After this process has been carried out, I subsequently process and purify the cells before injecting them into their new position in the body. Because it is most probable that up to 50 per cent of the transferred cells will not survive for longer than a few months, I "overfill" the relevant area. For example, if the area requires 20 mls of fat, I will fill it with 30–40 mls to allow for the loss.

The individual's own fatty cells are the best living filler since they are completely biocompatible and non-allergenic. This brings a lot of comfort and peace of mind to most of my patients.

Biceps and triceps implant procedures are performed under a general anaesthesia. I start the procedure by making an incision in the natural crease in the inner aspect of the upper arm, in what is known as the bicipital groove. It is the best place for the scar, as it tends to fade with time.

I then shape a "pocket" into which the implant is inserted and carefully positioned, inside the upper arm soft tissue area and muscle area. I then place a small dressing over the incision. I do not use tubigrip or crepe bandages. The patient can typically see the changes immediately after surgery.

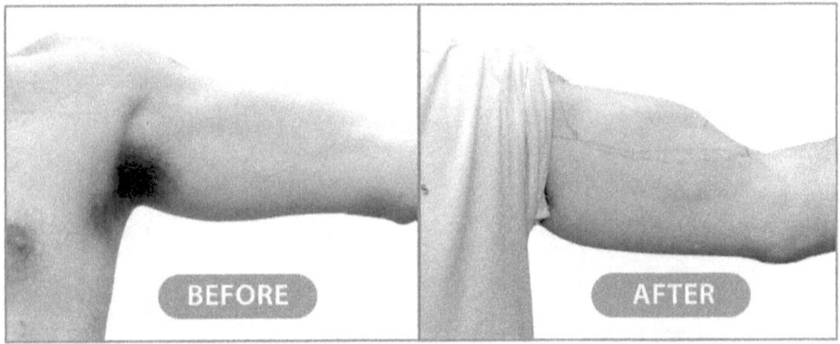

The photo is directly before and two hours after enhancing the patient's biceps and triceps with fat injections.

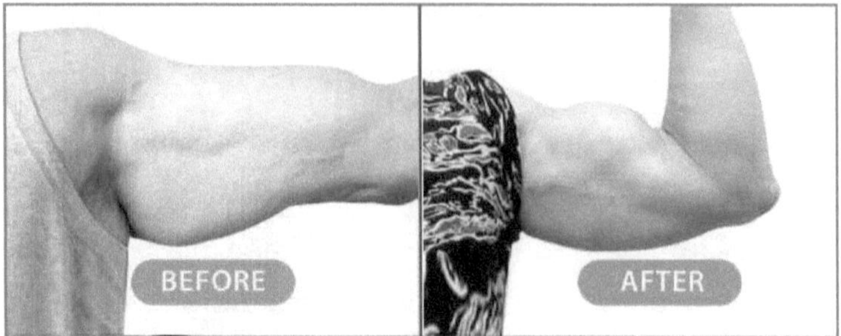

Before and after biceps and triceps enhancement.

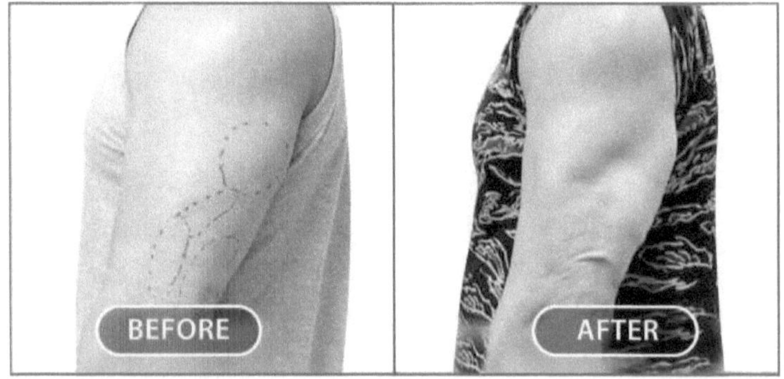

Notice the triceps area has been enhanced with a silicone implant.

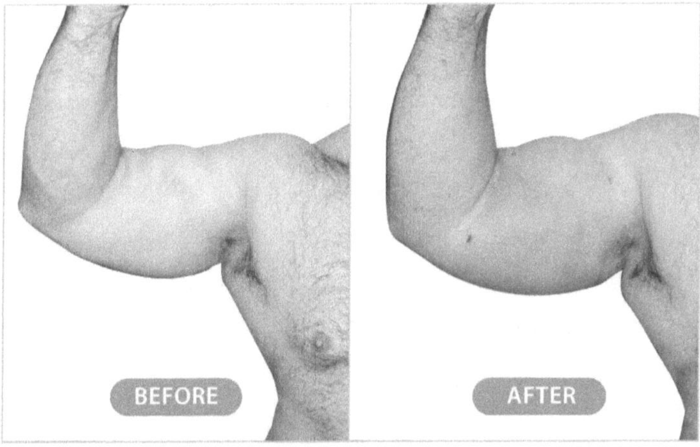

Before surgery, the patient had a noticeable contour deformity in the biceps area. The after photo is one hour after fat injections to his biceps and triceps to correct the deformities.

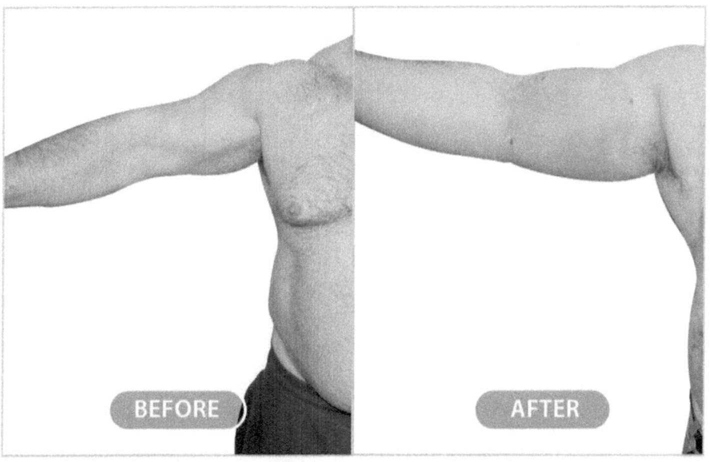

In the after photo, the injected biceps and triceps are bruised and swollen. The patient has maintained 60 per cent of the injected fat.

Calf Augmentation

Andy had always joked about his "chicken legs". The 35-year-old pro surfer and aspiring model was told time and time again that he had to "do something" about his skinny calves if he was going to break into catalog modelling. No matter how much he worked out, while the rest of his body developed muscles, his calves remained stick-like and skinny.

To boost his modelling career, Andy decided to have calf implants. The look he wanted was sculpted, but not overly so (as in the case of a bodybuilder). He just wanted a look that was in line with his chosen sport and his chosen profession. I used two small silicone implants that were placed beneath the inner aspect of the calf.

Not long after the implants, Andy booked a photoshoot. He sent the images off to his agent and was quickly booked for a prestigious menswear catalog!

Calf implants, or calf augmentation, is a plastic surgery procedure that is designed to increase the volume and enhance the shape of the calf area.

Both men and women find rounded calves attractive. I usually see men who are wanting to increase their muscle bulk and give them a more masculine look, whereas women wish to improve the symmetrical appearance of their legs.

Bodybuilders often report significant difficulties in building their calf muscles and seek calf enlargement procedures to give their legs better proportions.

Plastic surgeons also use this procedure to correct other conditions, including congenital defects, polio, spina bifida, and clubfoot, when such conditions are associated with undeveloped calves.

Over the last 30 years, calf augmentation has gained worldwide popularity. It is typically performed by either fat transfer, using the patient's own fat, or by placing silicone calf implants over the muscles, on the inner aspect of the calf. Some people, such as bodybuilders, may require larger augmentation, and in these individuals, an implant may be placed on both the medial (inner) and lateral (outer) aspects of the calf.

I perform the surgery by making a fine incision at the back of the knee in the crease, where it is nicely hidden. I incise the skin, fat and fascia, which is a deep thick tissue layer. I then lift the fascia, creating a pocket to fit the designed implant exactly. The implants are inserted through a "No Touch" sterile technique to minimise the risk of skin contamination. I then close the pocket and repair the skin and subcutaneous tissue. The patient goes home on the day of surgery.

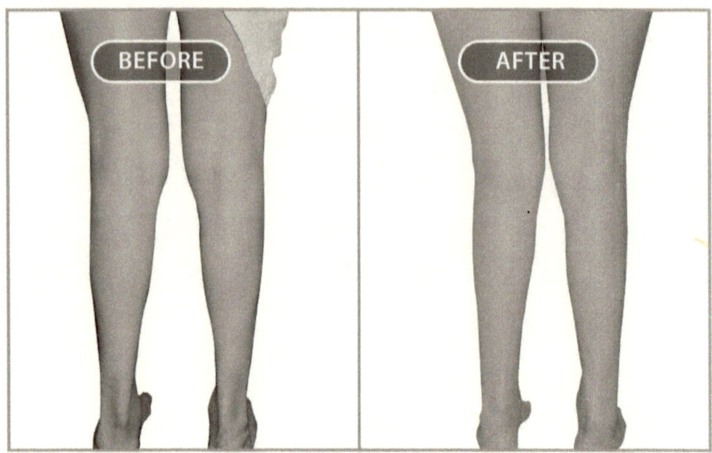

For patients born with muscle atrophy of the lower extremities, fat injections are the best choice for enhancement.

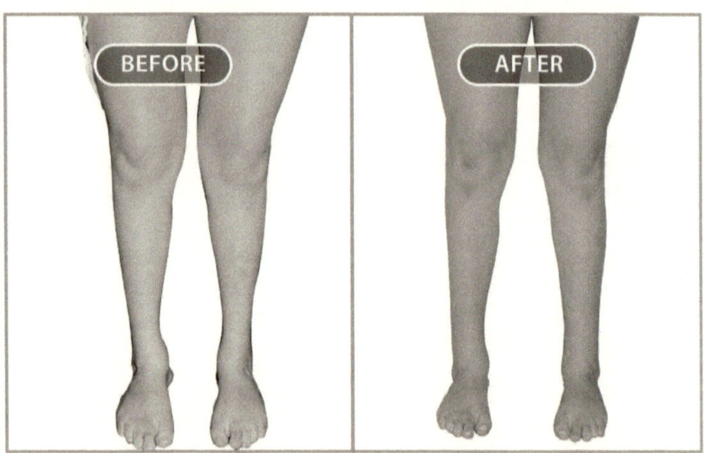

This is the same patient before and after her calf and ankle enhancement with fat injections.

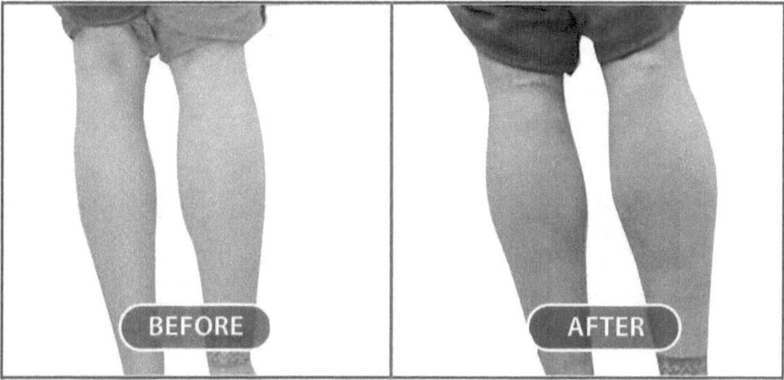

Natural calf augmentation using symmetrical implants.

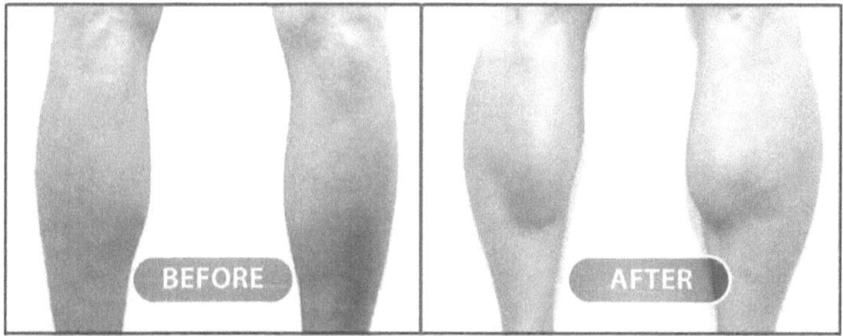

Fake-looking calf augmentation.

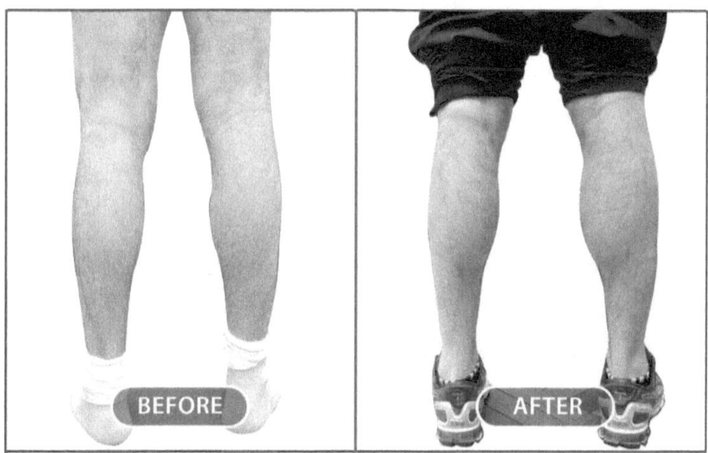

Calf augmentation with silicone implants.

Male Genital Surgery

For many men, the size and shape of their penis and scrotum is tremendously important to their sexual confidence. For men who were born with small or curved penises or feel that their testes are too small or are missing, there are several surgical procedures that can restore their self-confidence.

It is not uncommon for a man to feel insecure about the size and girth (thickness) of his penis. He may feel inhibited during sexual relations and/or be distressed by situations linked to swimming or sports. Most patients want a penis enlargement, not because they think their penis is too small when erect, but because it is too short while at rest (flaccid position); a condition known as "locker room syndrome".

Penis lengthening and/or thickening surgery is known as phalloplasty. This is a relatively new field in aesthetic surgery; however, this type of operation has become more popular.

The medical terminology for a short and thin penis is a "micropenis". There are many underlying causes for a short penis, so I use different manoeuvres to address each specific issue. This includes procedures to change and improve the appearance of the penis.

The suspensory ligament may require full division if the patient has a micropenis. The mons pubis may need to be reduced, liposucked or lifted if the underlying problem is a "buried penis". If too much skin was removed during circumcision, an additional skin graft or a VY advancement may be required. Some patients with a tight foreskin require surgery in two stages. The first procedure involves excision of the tight foreskin band and the second stage is phalloplasty.

Scientific guidelines must be followed when addressing the functional and potentially complex condition of the micropenis. It is also important to know that some patients have a normal sized penis but suffer from a psychological condition termed "penile dysmorphophobia". Surgery is not indicated for this group of patients.

Penis Lengthening Surgery

An extension of the penis can be achieved by loosening the ligament that suspends the penis inside the body, so the part of the penis that was inside the body is ejected and ends up on the outside.

Then, the erectile tissue is fastened to its new position, followed by inter-positioning of fatty tissue to further elongate and stabilise the penis during erection.

Finally, I advance the skin flap to further lengthen the skin of the penis at its base. This procedure does not affect the ability to achieve and maintain an erection. As long as no complications occur, the sensitivity of the skin and the head of the penis are not altered.

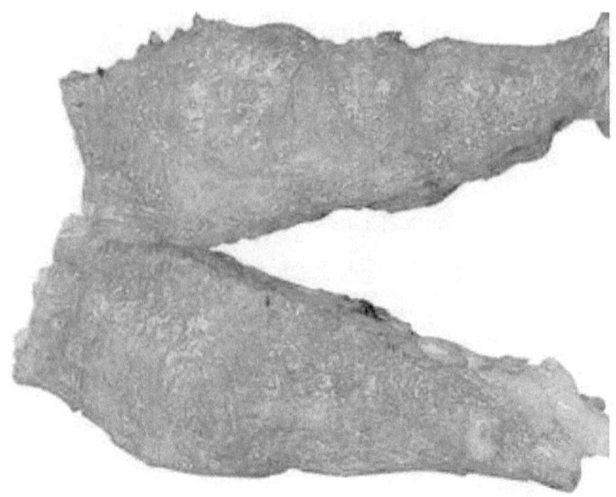

Dermal fat graft harvest. This is my preferable technique; I routinely use it for penis lengthening and girth increase. It produces an even surface and long-lasting results.

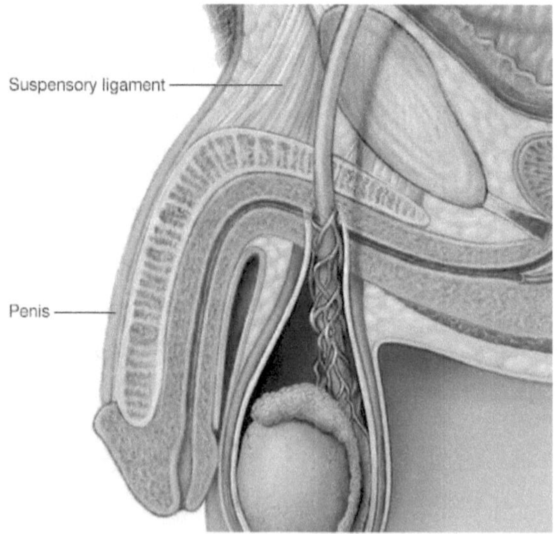

Division of the suspensory ligament alone is not enough to produce a satisfactory outcome. I routinely combine this penis lengthening procedure with fat injection, dermal fat grafting and/or a pubic lift.

Penis Thickening Surgery

The penile shaft is enlarged using a refined fat transplant technique. The fat is extracted from the pubic area, abdomen and waistline in a mini-liposuction procedure. I follow this with a fat purification process. Once blood and oil are removed from the fatty tissue, I inject the resulting fatty cells around the penis shaft through a tiny puncture hole. Typically, 20– 40 ml of fat is needed to fill the whole shaft of the penis. This procedure does not affect the patient's ability to achieve and maintain an erection.

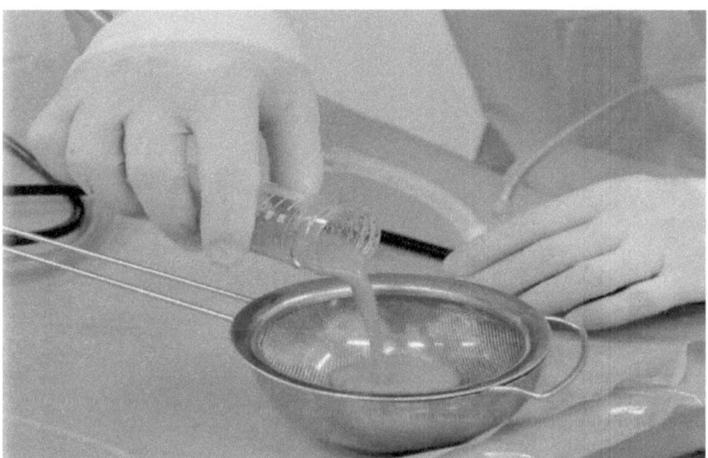

Purifying the harvested fat.

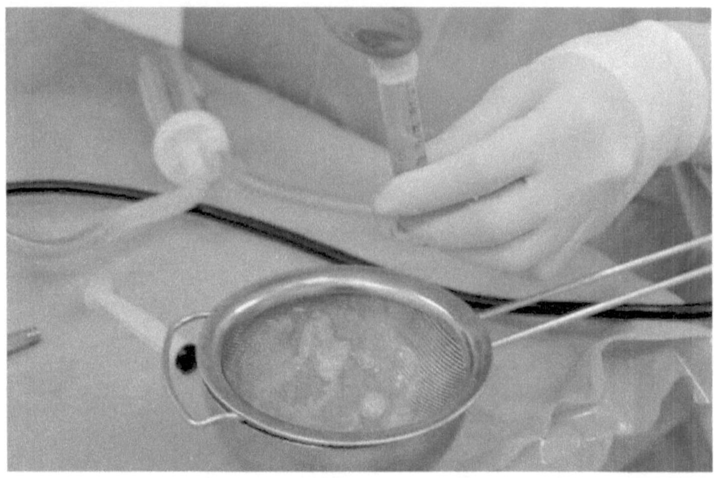

Fat preparation and transfer to syringes, ready to be used for augmentation.

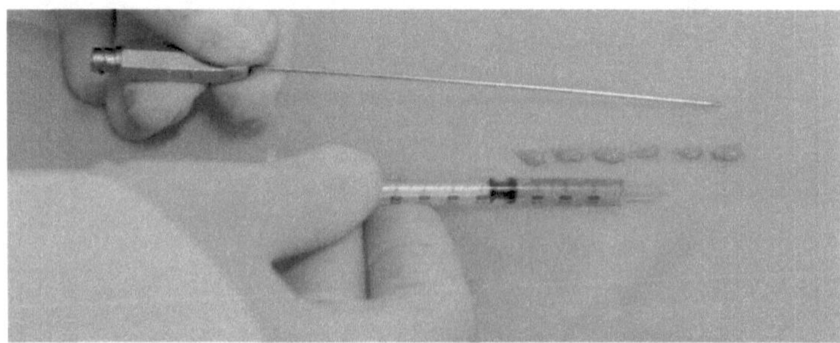

Here is a picture of the final product, refined cells. The best living filler is ready for injection.

Foreskin Surgery

Phimosis, or preputial stenosis, is a term that means any condition where the foreskin of the penis cannot be retracted. Most male infants are born with a foreskin that cannot be retracted, and the prepuce may be tight until after puberty. While it's usually painless, this condition can cause problems during intercourse or urination. Once phimosis is diagnosed, the available treatments include: topical corticosteroids, manual stretching, preputial plasty and circumcision.

Conservative treatments should be tried in the first instance and surgery as a second line of treatment. Several studies have shown that the application of topical steroids can safely and effectively treat phimosis in some cases. If such treatment is ineffective, several plastic surgery procedures are available for the treatment of phimosis, including:

- Preputial plasty is a minor surgical procedure performed as day surgery. It involves making a cut through the constrictive band of the foreskin, releasing the restricted band and closing the incision in a special way to prevent future constriction. This procedure allows the prepuce to be retained.

- Circumcision, which involves the removal of the tight foreskin band.

Testicular Implants

Testicular enlargement or enhancement is a procedure that is indicated for men who have:

- Atrophic (very small) testicles;

- No testicles (born with none or one testicle; or one or two undescended testicles; or the testicles have been removed because of trauma, disease or cancer);

- Asymmetrical testicles, i.e. one testicle is larger than the other.

Testicular implants are used to enhance testicular size or to balance the size of one testicle with the other testicle.

The best procedure to fill the scrotum is using testicular implants, which are ovoid in shape and soft in consistency. The objective of this surgery is to produce two well-represented testicles with pleasing contours.

Atrophic testes may still produce testosterone and sperm and should not be removed unless there are substantial medical indications to do so.

Ovoid testicular prostheses are available in both saline-filled and soft silicone models. The texture of the soft silicone models is minimally firmer than a normal testicle and generally well accepted. The implants come in different sizes, but generally, they are large, medium and small. Custom-made prostheses are also available but are more expensive.

I do not recommend very large testicular implants as they appear distinctly unnatural, dwarf the penis and may even reduce the depth of penetration during intercourse.

Testicular implant surgery is done as day surgery under general anaesthesia. I make a small incision in the front part of the scrotum and expose the internal aspect of the scrotal sack. I then insert the testicular prosthesis or implants in the dedicated sac. Following the placement of the prosthesis or testicular implant, the scrotal soft tissue and skin is closed in three layers.

Due to the elasticity of scrotal skin, the incision areas are hidden in the skin folds and the final scar is barely noticeable.

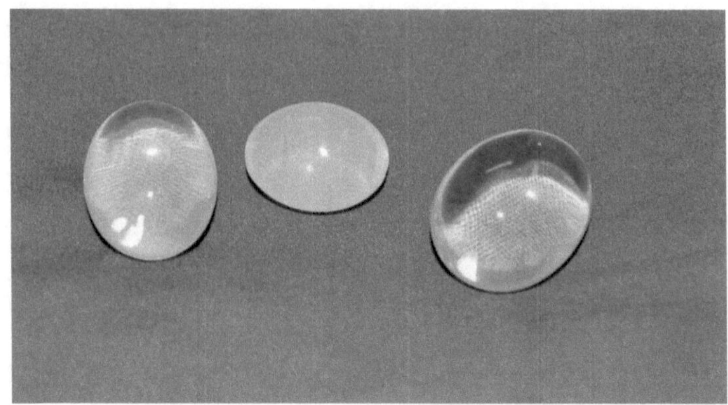

These are the types of testicular implants I commonly use: soft silicone and solid soft silicone elastomer.

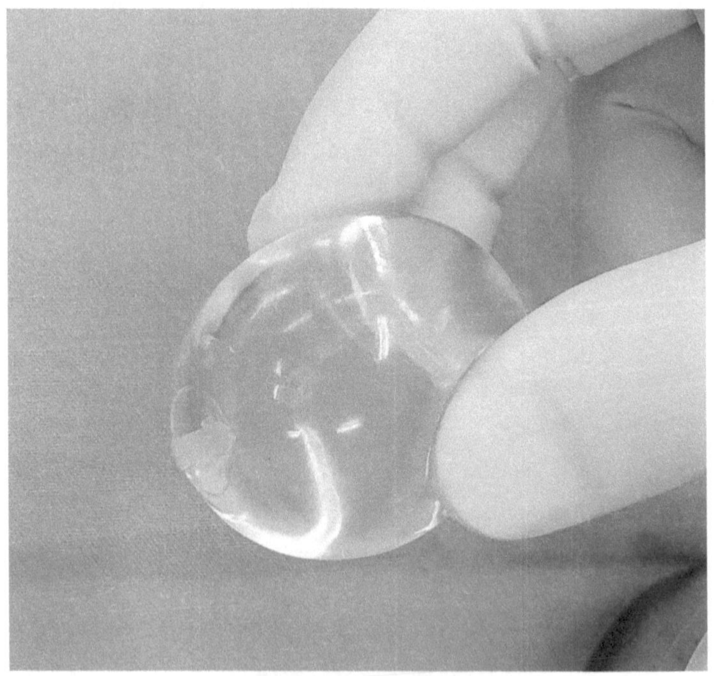

Soft silicone testicular implant.

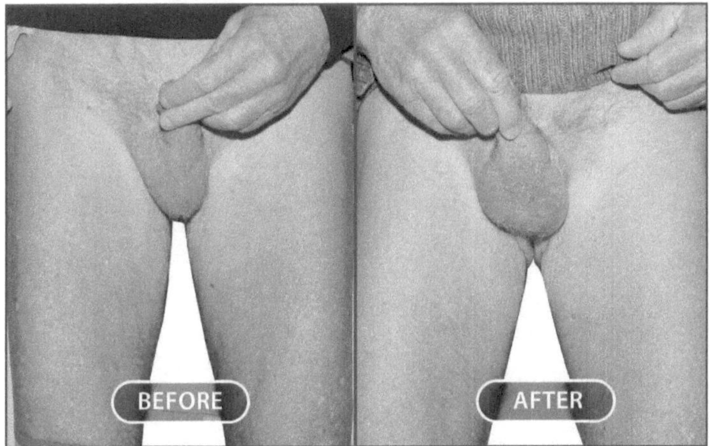

Right testicular implant surgery.

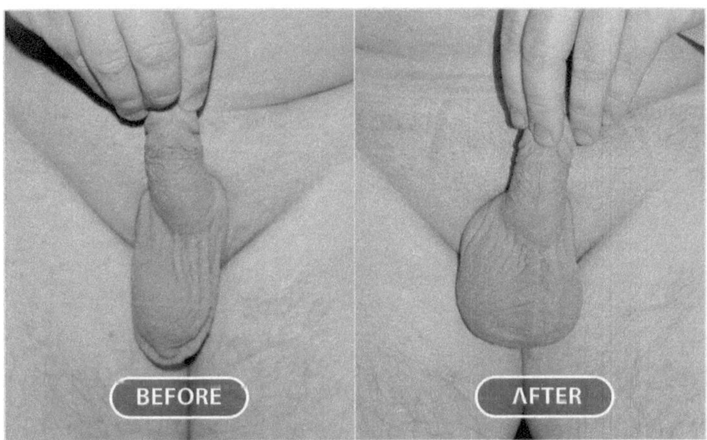

Left testicular implant surgery.

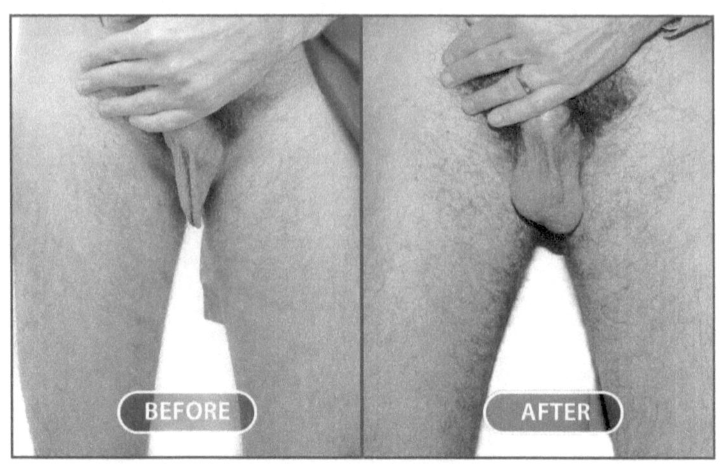

Bilateral testicular implant surgery.

CHAPTER SEVEN

Asian Plastic Surgery

Because Asian soft tissues, bony structures and skin are different from Caucasians, Asian plastic surgery deserves its own section.

Asian Eyelid Surgery

Anatomically, the difference between Asian and Caucasian eyelids is the position of the eyelid fold. The Asian eyelid typically starts at the crease very close to the eyelashes. As the crease becomes further away from the nose, it gets larger and larger until the midpoint of the pupil, at which point the fold runs parallel to the eyelash origin.

A Caucasian lid crease is slightly different in both shape and size. It typically tapers closer to the eyelashes as the fold goes out laterally so that it is more of an upside-down "U" shape, rather than a parallel shape to the eyelash lid. The Caucasian lid crease is also about 20 per cent larger than an Asian eyelid crease. The purpose of surgery is to create a natural-looking eyelid crease.

Many Asian people do not have a fold in the area above the eyelashes. It is possible to create an eyelid fold in a procedure called Asian blepharoplasty (eyelid surgery). The objective of the procedure is to create a natural-looking crease.

Other features of Asian eyelids that can be enhanced and/or corrected by plastic surgery include:

- A single eyelid called a Mongolian fold (excess skin/fold in the inner eyelid);

- Puffy upper and/or lower eyelids; and

- A thin appearance of the eyelids.

Popular Asian upper eyelid procedures include:

- Double eyelid surgery – supratarsal fold creation;

- Removal of excess skin – upper blepharoplasty;

- Ptosis repair – lazy eye surgery;

- Mongolian fold surgery – epicanthoplasty; and

- Big eye surgery – levator advancement surgery.

There are three surgical approaches to double eyelid surgery:

- Full incisional/scar;

- Partial incisional/scar; and

- No scar technique (durable suture technique).

Considerations include:

- The shape and characteristics of the eyelid;

- The amount of skin that needs to be removed;

- The amount of fat that needs to be trimmed;

- The type of eyelid shape that is desired; and

- Any previous history of eyelid procedures and eye conditions.

Four types of Asian eyelid surgery will be discussed in this section: 1) double eyelid surgery; 2) Mongolian fold surgery; 3) big eye surgery; and 4) lower eyelid surgery.

Double Eyelid Surgery

The traditional suture method used to create a natural crease, and hence the desired double eyelid, is a scarless and very popular procedure. It has significant advantages in terms of natural crease results, quick recovery and reproducibility (i.e. the ability of the surgeon to achieve a similar result for many procedures).

In the suture method, I create a crease by burying permanent non-reactive sutures (i.e. Prolene sutures, as used in heart valve surgery) and pinching a bit of the undersurface of the eyelid skin to the deep tissue. The procedure is performed under local anesthesia and takes 45 minutes. The healing time is a few days.

This other technique for creating an eyelid crease, known as the open approach, is reliable and known for its longevity. The drawbacks include a scar on the upper eyelid. However, this scar is in line with the fold and tends to fade with time. This approach is ideal for Asian patients who prefer a dramatic and deep crease.

The most natural shape of the fold is a tapered fold and the parallel fold, referring to the shape in relation to the margin of the inner half of the eyelid. The ideal size of the fold allows 2–3 mm of skin above the eyelashes to show on a direct frontal view with the eyes open. This also usually corresponds to a crease set at 7–8 mm from the lash line when the eyes are closed (with the skin on light tension).

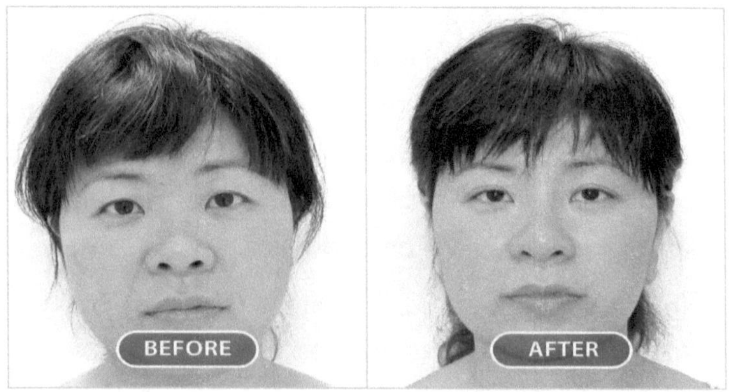

Asian blephararoplasty.

Mongolian Fold Surgery

Mongolian fold surgery, sometimes called medial epicanthoplasty, increases the visibility of the inner corners of the eye and reduces the distance between the eyes. The result is eyes that appear larger and closer together. For this reason, Mongolian fold surgery is a popular and uniquely Asian cosmetic surgery procedure.

The medial epicanthus is an excess fold of skin that covers the inner corner of the eyelid. It creates an illusion of a narrower eye and makes the eyes appear wider apart than they really are. The degree of severity ranges from non-existent or mild-to-moderate and then severe, depending on how much of the caruncle (the pink "bump" inside the eye corner) is exposed. Severe cases should be corrected; however, in the case of moderate skin folds, correction is optional.

One popular technique for correcting the fold is by augmenting the nose with a nasal implant as it takes some of the eyelid slackness away. Another option is repositioning the fold by what is known as a "jumping man flap" or "vy advancement flap" with a double opposing z-plasty technique.

Five essential factors for successful Mongolian fold surgery are:

1. The shape and characteristics of the Mongolian fold;

2. The amount of Mongolian fold that needs to be removed and repositioned;

3. Whether double eyelid surgery is requested at the same time;

4. The desired eyelid shape; and

5. Any previous history of eyelid procedures and eye conditions.

Big Eye Surgery

"Big eye surgery" is becoming more popular in Asian countries. Unlike Caucasians, Asian eyelid anatomy dictates smaller eye dimensions. Double eyelid surgery and Mongolian Fold correction surgery does make the eyes appear bigger and more open, but they do not actually increase the dimension of the eyes, and the eyes may still appear small. In this selected group of patients, big eye surgery can help, by actually increasing the size of the eye-opening.

Big eye surgery shortens and tightens the upper lid opening mechanism via a muscle called the levator. The job of the levator muscle is to raise up the eyelid. As the levator in the eyelid is shortened and tightened, the upper eyelid margins are pulled more open. Hence, the eyelid is rested at a more opened position and more of the eye is visible.

Lower Eyelid Surgery

Muscle weakness, excess fatty tissue and lax skin are some of the factors that lead to baggy lower eyelids in some people of Asian extraction.

There are two solutions to the problem:

- Non-surgical lower eyelid rejuvenation – skin tightening is achieved by laser or peel and volume restoration of the eyelid is achieved by soft tissue fillers or fat injection.

- Surgical lower eyelid rejuvenation – the excess fat is removed or redistributed through a small incision, which is hidden on the inside surface of the eyelid or just under the eyelashes.

Asian eyelids are sometimes characterised by a "severe form" of lower eye bags directly resulting from excess fatty tissue. Dark circles can also appear from a relatively young age. For this reason, eye bag removal is a popular Asian cosmetic procedure in all age groups. Lower eyelid surgery for wrinkle removal and skin tightening tends to be more popular in middle age and older patients.

The two most popular lower eyelid procedures are lower eyelid bag removal and lower eyelid skin tightening and wrinkle removal.

There are two surgical approaches involving lower eyelid bag removal:

- Internal approach – a small incision is made inside the lower eyelid (no visible external scar) and fat is removed through this incision.

- External approach – an incision is made just under the eyelashes and fat can be removed through this incision. Also loosened muscle can be tightened and the excess skin can be trimmed and tightened.

Lower eyelid skin tightening and wrinkle removal can be achieved by a surgical and a non-surgical approach, with a peel or laser. The non-surgical, or soft, approach to lower eyelid skin tightening, produces a great outcome in many cases.

Asian Facial Surgery

After eight years of caring for her terminally ill husband, while maintaining a full-time job, Tai's face showed the strain she had been under. She was 54, but her face looked much older. She had developed deep frown lines, bags under her eyes and the corners of her mouth were perpetually turned downward. There had simply been no time for the caregiver to take care of herself.

After her husband passed away, Tai wondered if she would ever find love again and someone with whom to spend her "golden years".

"Not with this face," she thought. "Who would want a face that has been so deeply etched by stress and sorrow?"

Tai chose to take care of herself, and she began with something she had never dared consider previously: a facelift. Emerging from years of caregiving into taking care of herself was like setting a butterfly free.

Tai's eyes regained their mischievous sparkle, and she started to smile again (most notably at her reflection in the mirror).

Facelift

Unlike Caucasian skin, Asian skin tends to be thicker and has less of a tendency for sagginess. For this reason, Asian patients requesting a facial rejuvenation procedure generally require a minimally invasive facelift.

The latest approach to facial rejuvenation entails more than just tightening of the skin and deep tissue. It is a comprehensive strategy to create a youthful appearance. It involves a facelift designed to minimise scarring, plus skin resurfacing, targeted liposuction, volumetric restoration, laser, TCA peel and other synergistic facelift procedures.

The 21st-century approach to enhancing facial beauty emphasises the importance of shifting and restoring facial volumes rather than only tightening the skin and deep tissue.

Different techniques are available for Asian facelifts:

- Facial Volumetric Restoration — also known as face fat injection. Fat is removed from the areas of excess fat, such as the neck, and then injected into areas that do not have enough fat, such as the cheeks.

- Face Lift — more advanced facial sagginess may require a more significant and effective lifting technique involving repositioning and tightening of underlying facial soft tissues and removing the excess and redundant skin. This is also known as the S lift, MACS lift, or short scar facelift.

- Neck Lift — like the facelift, the neck can be lifted. The scars can be hidden behind the ears.

- Soft Face Lift — a soft-facelift in Asian patients is typically performed in a minimally invasive manner through skin peel, laser treatment, face fat injection and neck liposuction.

- Jaw reduction — many Asian patients have a broad lower part of the face due to either a large jawbone or large musculature in the area. A prominent jawline tends to be out of proportion to the rest of the face. The enlarged or masculine jawline can be made to look more feminine and slender in one of two ways:

» The first is a surgical approach that "shaves" the jaw to reduce the outer portion of the jaw with the result of narrowing the face.

» The second more common approach is to non-surgically narrow the masseter muscle (a facial muscle that plays an important role in chewing food). This involves an injection of Botox (botulinum toxin) into the muscle on both sides of the jaw. It is a safe and effective treatment, performed in the office on the day of the consultation. It produces immediate results that last for six months. It is recommended that this procedure is repeated every six-to-nine months.

Asian Brow Lift

A brow lift is just one of the procedures that can help Asian patients achieve a younger look. At around age 30, some people develop what appears to be an excess of upper eyelid skin. The reason for this apparent excess skin is often sagging of the eyebrow and forehead. The ideal procedure to correct this sagging skin is a brow lift, which I typically perform through an incision within the hairline.

During the brow lift procedure, I make one incision on each side in the scalp. Through this incision, I work my way down to the eyebrow and lift it. This elevates the lateral brow area so that there is a slight arch to the brow. The central portion does not get lifted because this can lead to a "surprised" expression.

Facial Implants

Facial implants are a popular Asian cosmetic surgery. Unlike Caucasians, Asian people have foreheads, chins and midfaces that are naturally set back. Enhancement of these structures results in attractive facial features that project further and give the patient a more harmonious facial contour.

There are numerous plastic surgery implant and enhancement procedures available for Asian patients, including:

- Facial Implants – using silicone implants, Medpore implants, or Gortex implants. As the incision is made through the mouth, the scar is hidden. There is about a week of post-surgery downtime.

- Injections with soft tissue fillers – they can be permanent or temporary. There is no downtime.

- Fat/stem cell injections into the forehead, cheek and chin. This is very a popular technique as it produces no facial scarring.

Asian Liposuction

Liposuction is used to remove stubborn pockets of fat that are not responsive to diet and exercise. On Asian patients, the arms and waist tend to be the areas that collect fat. Other areas that may require liposuction are the calves, the inner and outer thighs, and the back. However, due to the tendency of Asian patients to scar more easily, I pay particular attention to avoid any unfavourable scars during liposuction.

I often perform Asian liposuction under general anaesthesia with the tumescent technique, which involves injecting a mixture of local anaesthetic, adrenaline and saline just below a patient's skin. The anaesthetic numbs the skin while the adrenaline constricts blood vessels. The advantage of this technique is that there is very little bruising and pain after the procedure.

Liposuction is performed as day surgery, so patients go home on the day of the procedure. Most people who receive this type of liposuction can get back to their normal routines and work in just a couple of days.

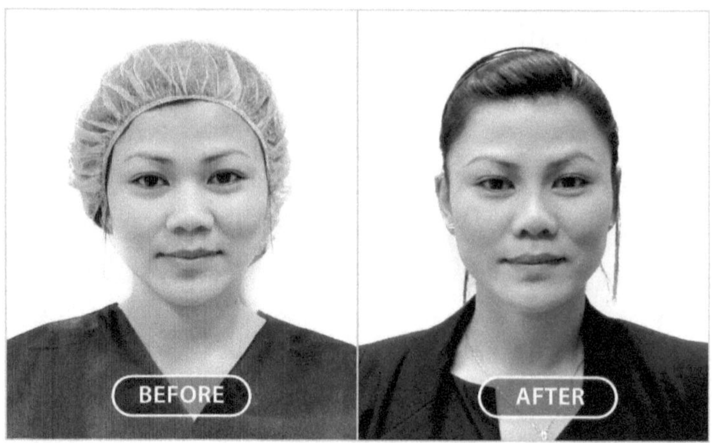

This patient had Asian rhinoplasty, including the insertion of a nasal implant.

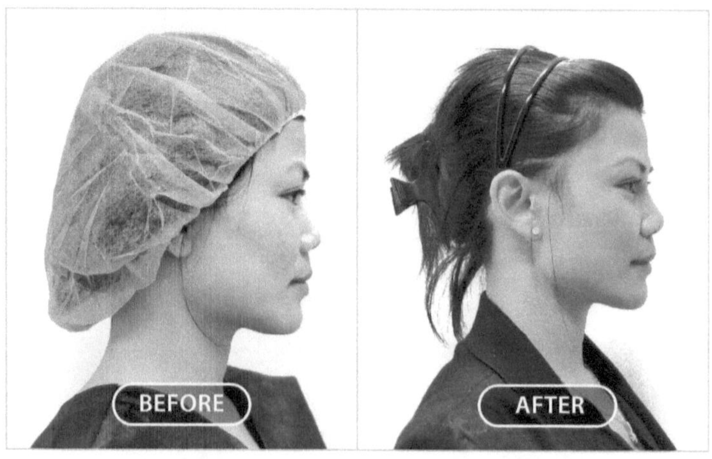

Notice the projected bridge of the nose.

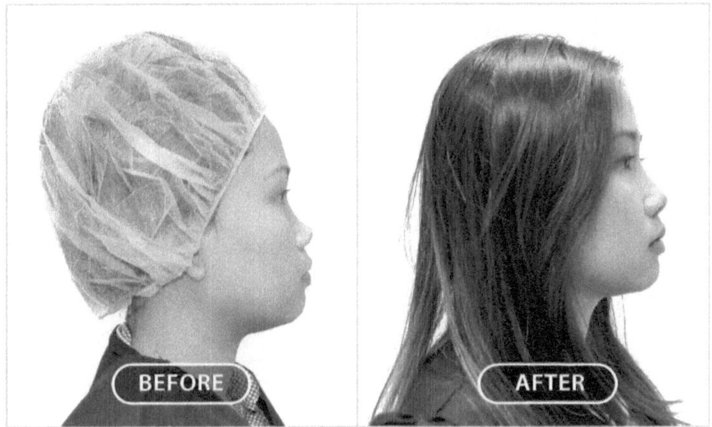

Augmentation rhinoplasty with a nasal implant.

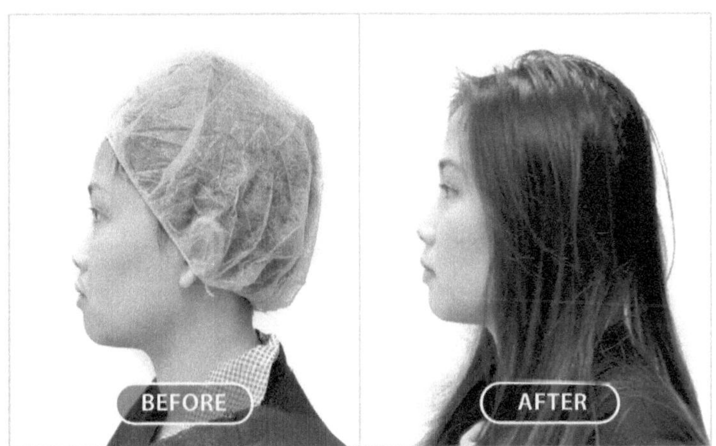

Notice the improved profile.

Keloid Scar Removal

Keloid scars are wide, purple or brown-colored raised scars that can result from infections, bad wound healing, harsh tissue handling, improper suturing techniques and/ or genetic predisposition.

Certain anatomic areas – such as the middle of the chest, sternum, shoulders and ear lobes – are more prone to keloid scarring than other anatomic areas. Patients of Asian and African descent are genetically predisposed to keloid and hypertrophic scarring.

There are a number of treatments for keloid scarring including: steroid injection, surgical intralesional excision, pressure technique, hydration therapy, silicone sheet (sica care sheet) and radiotherapy.

I customise the treatment to the width and anatomic position of the patient's scar. Commonly, patients require a combination of the above treatments for the minimisation and management of their keloid scars.

CONCLUSION

As someone who keenly observes how humans age (myself included), I'm intrigued to learn about every method available that can safely and reliably help people maintain and improve their looks and body.

I love what I do and find it very satisfying to improve my patients' lives through plastic surgery. I'm passionate about safety as well as medical and surgical expertise. And, as my attention to detail will attest, I have developed a finely tuned eye for natural beauty.

It is my desire to soften the effects of ageing in my patients. Life is stressful enough as it is. If I can provide my patients with a more rested and happier look … If I can help them increase their satisfaction with their bodies and improve their quality of life … If I can help them achieve their goals when it comes to their appearance and physique, then I have done my job.

My final advice is not to rush into surgery, but instead take your time and think about what surgery can and cannot do for you. Planning for surgery is the most crucial part. Do not worry about the smallest details of techniques; that is the job of your plastic surgeon. Rather, prepare yourself for your recovery period, which may be unpleasant and take from two days to four weeks depending on the surgical procedure.

Also remember that you are doing the surgery for yourself – to improve your physical appearance and boost your confidence – not for others.

Good luck on your journey to a new you!

Dr Laith Barnouti

SPECIALIST PLASTIC SURGEON, FRACS
CONJOINT SENIOR LECTURER, UNIVERSITY OF NSW
SYDNEY, AUSTRALIA

"The secret ingredient is always love…"

—Patrick Tonnard, MD, PHD

SPECIALIST PLASTIC SURGEON GENT,
BELGIUM